The EMT Handbook of Emergency Care

The EMT Handbook of Emergency Care

D.J. ARNESON
B.A., E.M.T.-IV

MAUREEN L. BRUCE
R.N., B.S.N., M.A., C.A.S., E.M.T.-IV
EMS Instructor, State of Connecticut

Illustrations by **Lee Berliner**

Philadelphia   **J.B. LIPPINCOTT COMPANY**

London · Mexico City · New York · St. Louis · São Paulo · Sydney

"We love the things we love for what they are."
Robert Frost

Dave, Matthew, and Mark
M. L. B.

Bea, Leif, and Marc
D. J. A.

Sponsoring Editor: Patricia Cleary
Manuscript Editor: Virginia Barishek
Indexer: D. J. Arneson
Design Director: Tracy Baldwin
Design Coordinator: Don Shenkle
Designer: Adrianne Onderdonk Dudden
Production Supervisor: Kathleen Dunn
Production Coordinator: Susan Hess
Compositor: Bi-Comp, Incorporated
Printer/Binder: R. R. Donnelley & Sons Company

Library of Congress Cataloging-in-Publication Data

Arneson, D. J.
    The EMT handbook of emergency care.

    Includes index.
    1. Emergency medicine—Handbooks, manuals, etc.
2. First aid in illness and injury—Handbooks, manuals,
etc. 3. Emergency medical technicians—Handbooks,
manuals, etc. I. Bruce, Maureen L. II. Title.
RC86.8.A76   1987   616'.025   86-7404
ISBN 0-397-54595-9

The authors and publisher have exerted every effort to ensure that
drug selection and dosage set forth in this text are in accord with
current recommendations and practice at the time of publication.
However, in view of ongoing research, changes in government
regulations, and the constant flow of information relating to drug
therapy and drug reactions, the reader is urged to check the package
insert for each drug for any change in indications and dosage and for
added warnings and precautions. This is particularly important when
the recommended agent is a new or infrequently employed drug.

Preface

The EMT Handbook of Emergency Care is a comprehensive digest of current basic life support (BLS) data presented in a step-by-step format for immediate reference.

Your ability as an EMT is not measured by what you carry with you in a book but by what you can recall at the instant of need. However, the range of skills and the amount of information an EMT must know to provide BLS services is impressive, and very few are likely to know it all. It is the aim of this manual to be an adjunct to what you already know, not to replace it.

Your skills as an EMT are constantly being refreshed by experience in the field, in-service training, study, reading, and review. This manual is designed to help you in each as a source of accurate information.

On the other hand, *The EMT Manual of Emergency Care* is not a textbook or a "how-to" book, and it should not be used as such. It is a manual of condensed information written expressly for trained EMTs who already know the procedures referred to and who are familiar with BLS delivery.

The range of BLS protocols across the nation is extensive; no manual could hope to include them all. In any matter where local protocol conflicts with the information in this book, follow your local protocol.

Most important of all, though you are responsible for the decisions you make, you do not have to make them alone. Whenever you are uncertain about what to do, request assistance from your medical control; their advice is yours for the asking.

As a practical matter, the information in this manual applies to standard situations. But as you know, no patient, run, illness, or accident is the same as any other. Treat each situation as a one-of-a-kind event and every patient as unique and adjust your care accordingly.

D. J. Arneson
Maureen L. Bruce

Acknowledgments

This manual's value to you and to your patients has been immensely increased by the encouragement, effort, and expertise of many people.

Every EMT experiences at one time or another the sense of helplessness that comes when faced with an impossible call. And all EMTs know the welcome relief when assistance arrives at last. Whether it's an ambulance crew member at the scene or the voice of the ER physician on the radio, the knowledge that you are not alone often lets you get the job done.

We were not alone either when researching and writing this manual. Many helped. We acknowledge their help here so that you and they will know its significance to this work, and to yours.

We are grateful to the following for their medical, technical, and personal assistance. Their expertise has contributed accuracy and excellence to this manual to make our job and yours easier.

Medical Consultants

Alice D. Cupole, R.N., B.S.N., EMT, School Nurse, Newtown Public Schools, Newtown, CT; Oxford, CT Ambulance Association

Thomas F. Draper, M.D., Director of Pediatric Ambulatory Care, Danbury Hospital, Danbury, CT

Gerald J. Germano, M.D., Department of Pediatrics, Griffin Hospital, Derby, CT; Yale–New Haven Hospital, New Haven, CT

Salvatore Iannotti, M.D., Chairman of the Department of Obstetrics and Gynecology, Griffin Hospital, Derby, CT; Assistant Professor, Yale University School of Nursing, New Haven, CT

Dennis Pilarczyck, M.D., Attending Physician, Emergency Department, Waterbury Hospital, Waterbury, CT

Marietta G. Sonido, M.D., Clinical Director Medical/Surgical Services, Fairfield Hills Hospital, Newtown, CT

Romeo A. Sonido, M.D., Emergency Department Physician, Griffin Hospital, Derby, CT

Ronald Tietjen, M.D., Attending Physician, Orthopedic Surgery, Danbury Hospital, Danbury, CT; Clinical Attending Physician in Orthopedics, Columbia–Presbyterian Medical Center, New York, NY; Director, Western Connecticut Sports Medicine Clinic, Danbury, CT

Anthony G. Wayne, M.D., Department of Pediatrics, Griffin Hospital, Derby, CT; Yale–New Haven Hospital, New Haven, CT

Technical and Personal Assistance

Beatrice Arneson, M.S., Regional Director, Connecticut Community Care, Inc., Waterbury, CT

Lee Berliner, medical illustrator, Newtown, CT

David Bruce, B.S., EMT, Oxford Ambulance Association, Oxford, CT

Robert Corrigan, Emergency Medical Services Instructor, State of Connecticut; EMT, Southbury, CT Ambulance Association

Elmer J. Sunyog, Flambeau Products Corp., Middlefield, OH

Epson Computers; Epson America, Inc., Torrance, CA

Valdocs+ Computer Software; Rising Star Industries, Torrance, CA

The complex task of data management and manuscript production was made possible by an Epson computer using Valdocs+ software.

And a special thank you to our editor, Patricia Cleary, for her vision and her encouragement to write this manual.

Introduction

"An expert is one who knows more and more about less and less."

Nicholas Murray Butler, American educator

The constantly growing body of knowledge required by EMTs to provide professional pre-hospital emergency care is an example of the need for specialization in today's world, that is, the need to be an expert.

Technology, techniques, and standards are ever changing. To stay current, a dedicated EMT must remain abreast of those changes *and* maintain certified proficiency through in-service training, refresher courses, and exams.

Expertise in Basic Life Support is demanding; Advanced Life Support is more so. EMTs who want to upgrade to advanced levels require a body of knowledge that seems staggering at times, particularly for new, volunteer, part-time, low-frequency, and other pre-hospital care providers whose primary occupation is not emergency care.

Competence at every level of emergency care from newly certified EMT to seasoned ER physician requires mastery of fundamentals—the basics.

The EMT Handbook of Emergency Care is a digest of essential BLS data tightly organized into a comprehensive manual for instant reference by trained personnel at the EMT-A level and above. Although its use is self defining, some simple guidelines will increase its utility.

The EMT Handbook of Emergency Care is not a textbook. It may be used to supplement standard EMT texts for study and review, but it is not meant to replace them.

The EMT Handbook of Emergency Care is not a "how-to" book. The intended user is a certified EMT who already knows how to provide Basic Life Support.

The information and procedures outlined herein are for reference as adjuncts to the user's training and knowledge, not as substitutes for them.

Use of this book to assess, diagnose, treat, or provide care of any kind to any person by unqualified personnel is expressly outside its purpose and constitutes misuse of its contents.

The EMT Handbook of Emergency Care is not intended for use as a "checklist" to substitute for learned skills. Although it may be a helpful reference at any time, it should not replace the judgment or training of its user or any protocol, guideline, or directive the user is subject to.

In all instances, local protocols, guidelines, and directives supersede the material in this handbook.

Basic to all emergency care is the fact that no patient or call is exactly the same. Although the emergency care principles and procedures outlined in this handbook are consistent with standard teaching and training texts, their application depends entirely on the special circumstances of a given call. It is the responsibility of the EMT to consider every aspect of each call (location, mechanism of injury, weather, etc.) and patient (physical, emotional, medical, and other history) before providing care.

The recommended way to learn to use this handbook is to become familiar with the format and contents by browsing, and then to read each topic thoroughly. Periodic review will keep the data fresh in mind.

Information is grouped by sections listed in the table of contents. Topics within sections are listed on separate contents pages at the beginning of each section.

Essential BLS data for each topic is presented in separate two-page spreads identified at the top of the pages. The right-hand page consists of text condensed into the basics for instant reference. The left-hand page contains illustrations or additional text that supplements the material on the right.

Marginal reference words (Priority, Definition, Signs and Symptoms) identify the data to their left.

To find information, refer to the table of contents, the section contents pages, or the index for the page number of the topic you seek.

The data is presented in logical, consistent order whenever possible (head to toe, high to low priority, most to least common, alphabetized). However, because virtually all the essential information for a given topic is contained on a single (right-hand) page, some will be extraneous because it is rare for all data to apply to any one situation.

For example, a patient may not present *all* the signs and symptoms of Angina, and *all* the steps listed under Treatment for Soft Tissue injury may not be required to stabilize another patient. Therefore, no hard rule is implied by the order in which the data is presented or that it is included. It is up to the trained EMT to determine by thorough assessment and professional judgment which data applies in each situation.

That same judgment is to be used to request resource personnel such as medical control, police and fire departments, extrication assistance, burn, poison, disaster and radiation control units, and others.

Whether for instant access or casual review, *The EMT Handbook of Emergency Care* is designed to be *used.* It can be made even more useful by writing in local protocols, personal notes, new or updated material, and other information or changes (CPR standards, for example) specific to the EMT, region, or service, and this is recommended.

Every ambulance run, whether an emergency or not, is unique. The EMT responder—professional, volunteer, police officer, fireman, or other—has only one opportunity to carry out the training and skills required for each call. That one chance cannot be overvalued, and when the issue is life and death it is priceless.

Be an expert.

Contents

SECTION 5 Medical Emergencies 157

SECTION 6 Environmental Emergencies 207

SECTION 7 Pediatric/Obstetric Emergencies 237

SECTION 8 Psychological Emergencies 253

SECTION 9 Special Concerns 263

The EMT Handbook
of Emergency Care

SECTION 1

Anatomy/Physiology

This section reviews body structures, systems, and functions.

Standard terms promote efficient, effective patient assessment and care and enable accurate communication. They are used in this section and throughout the book.

Guidelines

1. Use standard medical terminology when communicating verbally or in writing with other health professionals.
2. Use everyday language when talking with patients or others who may not be familiar with medical terminology.
3. Develop proficiency by mentally observing and describing people around you in standard medical terms.

This section will help you to

1. Describe position and location of injuries on a patient
2. Position a patient for treatment and transport
3. Describe movement and position of jointed parts
4. Locate standard body reference points
5. Locate enclosed spaces and their organs
6. Locate the major bones in the body
7. Review major body systems, structures, organs, and functions

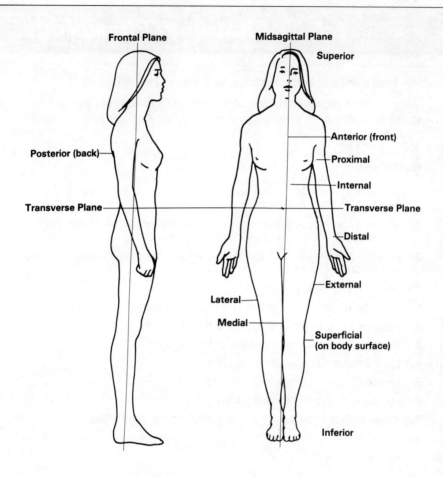

Topographic Anatomy

Universal medical terminology used to describe position and location on the body in anatomic position (standing erect, facing forward, arms down at sides, palms forward)   *Definition*

Midsagittal	Divides body into right and left halves	*Planes*
Transverse	Divides top from bottom at umbilicus	
Frontal	Divides front from back	

Anterior	Front	*Terms*
Posterior	Back	
Lateral	Away from midline	
Medial	Toward midline	
Proximal	Point on extremity nearest midline	
Distal	Point on extremity away from midline	
Superior	Toward the head	
Inferior	Toward the feet	
Internal	Inside the body	
External	Outside the body	
Superficial	Near or on body surface	

Right and *left* refer to the *patient's* right and left.   *Note*

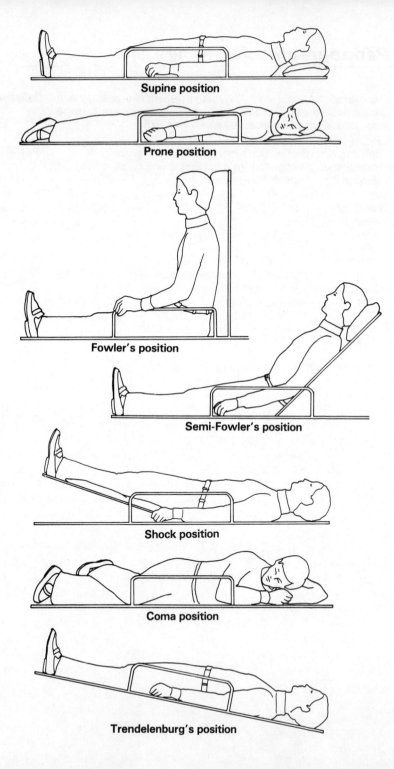

Supine position

Prone position

Fowler's position

Semi-Fowler's position

Shock position

Coma position

Trendelenburg's position

Patient Positions

Standard ways to place the body to facilitate treatment and transportation with minimum aggravation and maximum benefit to the patient and condition

Definition

Positions

Supine	Patient horizontal, on back
Prone	Patient horizontal, on stomach, head to side
Fowler's	Patient sitting upright, legs outstretched
Semi-Fowler's	Patient sitting at 45° angle, legs outstretched
Shock	Patient supine with feet elevated 8 to 12 in
Coma (left lateral recumbent)	Patient lying on left side, left knee and thigh flexed, head resting on left arm, facing down
Trendelenburg	Patient supine, head down, legs and torso raised to a 30° angle

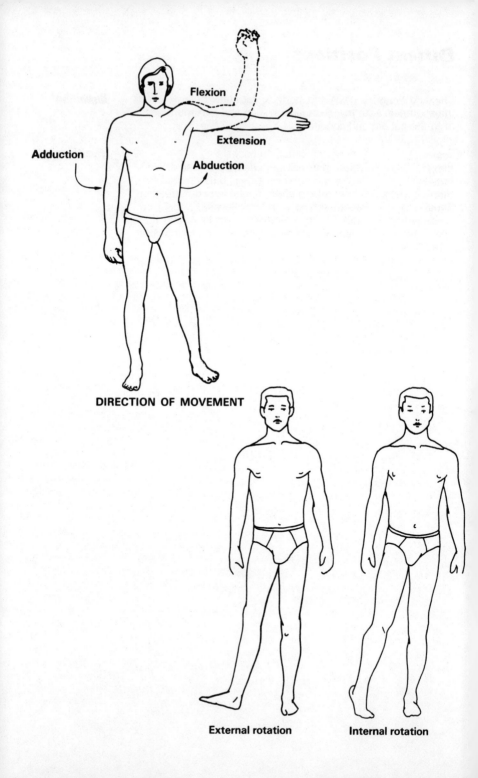

Flexion

Extension

Adduction

Abduction

DIRECTION OF MOVEMENT

External rotation

Internal rotation

Direction of Movement

The way jointed body parts can move and the relative positions in which they may be found on a patient — *Definition*

Abduction	Motion away from the midline	*Terms*
Adduction	Motion toward the midline	
Flexion	Bending (closing) a joint	
Extension	Straightening (opening) a joint	
Internal Rotation	Medial turning around a central axis	
External Rotation	Lateral turning around a central axis	

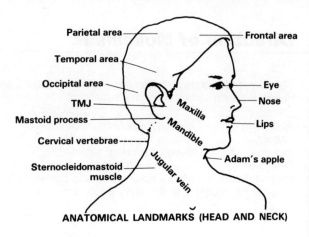

ANATOMICAL LANDMARKS (HEAD AND NECK)

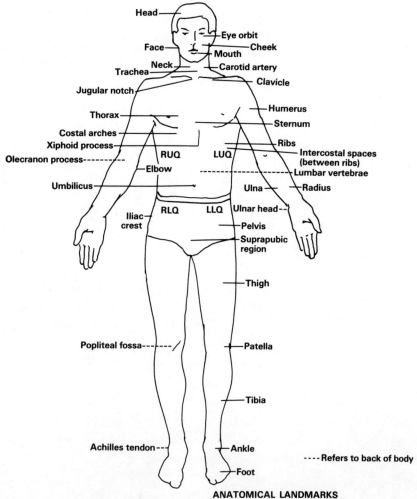

ANATOMICAL LANDMARKS

Anatomical Landmarks

Medically recognized bony prominences, muscle contours, blood vessels, lumps, depressions, and imaginary lines used as reference points on the body.

Definition

Location

Head
Cranium (skull)
  Frontal region
  Temporal region
  Parietal region
  Occipital region
  Mastoid process

Neck
Adam's apple
Trachea
Carotid artery
External jugular vein
Jugular notch
Sternocleidomastoid muscle
Cervical vertebrae

Face
  Supraorbital ridge
  Eye orbits
  Eyes
  Nose
  Cheeks (zygoma)
  Mouth
  Lips
  Upper jaw (maxilla)
  Lower jaw (mandible)
  Temporomandibular joint

Thorax (Chest)
Anterior
  Clavicle (collarbone)
  Sternum (breastbone)
  Xiphoid process
  Ribs (12)
  Intercostal spaces
  Costal arches

Posterior
  Scapula
  Thoracic vertebrae

Pelvis
Iliac crest
Pelvic bones
Suprapubic region
Lumbar vertebrae

Abdomen
Umbilicus
Right upper quadrant (RUQ)
Left upper quadrant (LUQ)
Right lower quadrant (RLQ)
Left lower quadrant (LLQ)

Lower Extremity
Thigh (femur)
Patella (kneecap)
Popliteal fossa
Tibia (shinbone)
Ankle; Achilles tendon
Foot

Upper Extremity
Upper arm (humerus)
Lower arm (radius/ulna)
Elbow
Olecranon (elbow)

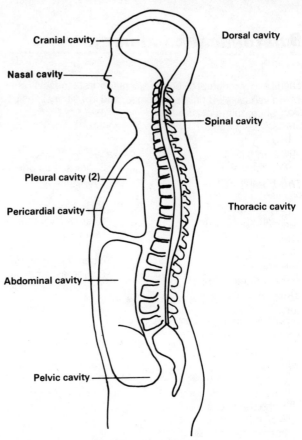

Cranial cavity

Dorsal cavity

Nasal cavity

Spinal cavity

Pleural cavity (2)

Pericardial cavity

Thoracic cavity

Abdominal cavity

Pelvic cavity

BODY CAVITIES

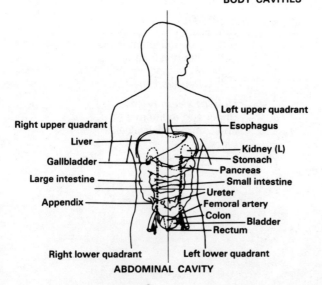

Left upper quadrant

Right upper quadrant

Esophagus

Liver

Kidney (L)

Gallbladder

Stomach

Pancreas

Large intestine

Small intestine

Appendix

Ureter

Femoral artery

Colon

Bladder

Rectum

Right lower quadrant

Left lower quadrant

ABDOMINAL CAVITY

Body Cavities

Enclosed spaces containing organs within the body   ***Definition***

Dorsal Cavity
Cranial cavity
  Brain
Spinal cavity
  Spinal cord

Nasal Cavity
Septum
Nasal fossae

Cavities

Thoracic Cavity
Pleural cavities (2)
  Lungs
Pericardial cavity
  Heart
Esophagus
Aorta
Vena cava

Buccal Cavity
Tongue
Teeth

Abdominal Cavity
Left upper quadrant
  Stomach
  Spleen
  Transverse colon
  Liver
  Left kidney
  Pancreas
Left lower quadrant
  Descending colon
  Small intestine
  Major artery and vein,
    left leg
  Abdominal aorta
  Ureter, left

Right upper quadrant
  Gallbladder
  Pancreas
  Transverse colon
  Liver
  Right kidney

Right lower quadrant
  Appendix
  Small intestine
  Major artery and vein,
    right leg
  Ureter, right

Pelvic Cavity
Bladder
Ureters
Rectum
Ovaries (female)
Uterus (female)

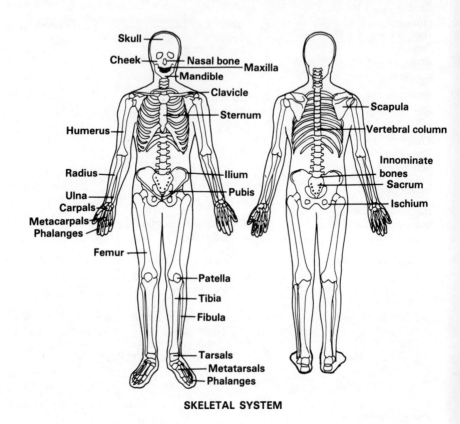

SKELETAL SYSTEM

Skeletal System

The major bones in the human body

Definition

Skull
Frontal
Temporal
Parietal
Occipital

Face
Nasal (nose)
Zygomatic (cheek)
Maxilla (upper jaw)
Mandible (lower jaw)

Spinal Column
Vertebrae
Sacrum
Coccyx (tailbone)

Thorax
Clavicle (collarbone)
Scapula (shoulder blade)
Sternum (breastbone)
Ribs

Pelvis
Innomiate bone
Ilium

Ischium
Pubis

Upper Extremity
Humerus (upper arm bone)
Radius (forearm bone)
Ulna (forearm bone)
Carpals (wrist bones)
Metacarpals (hand bones)
Phalanges (finger bones)

Lower Extremity
Femur (thigh bone)
Patella (kneecap)
Tibia (leg bone)
Fibula (leg bone)
Tarsals (ankle bones)
Metatarsals (foot bones)
Phalanges (toe bones)

There are 206 bones in the human body.

Note

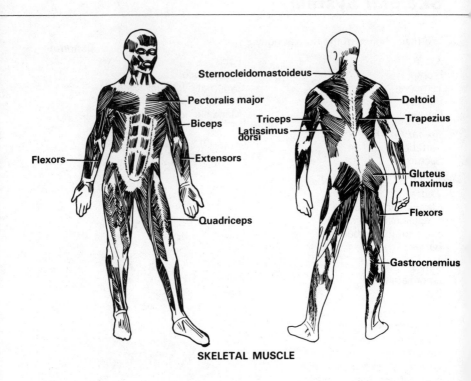

SKELETAL MUSCLE

Sternocleidomastoideus

Pectoralis major

Biceps

Flexors

Extensors

Quadriceps

Triceps

Latissimus dorsi

Deltoid

Trapezius

Gluteus maximus

Flexors

Gastrocnemius

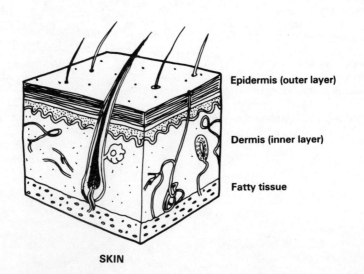

Epidermis (outer layer)

Dermis (inner layer)

Fatty tissue

SKIN

Muscular System and Skin

MUSCLE Richly vascular, elastic tissue made of fibers that contract to cause movement in body parts and organs, give the body shape, and form its walls
Definition and Function

STRIATED *Striated* muscles are attached to the skeleton.
Types

SMOOTH The muscular part of the visceral organs is composed of *smooth* muscle.

CARDIAC The muscle forming the heart is *cardiac* muscle.

Muscle cells
Blood vessels
Tendons (fibrous extensions that attach muscles to bones)
Components

Muscle tissue is always in a slight state of contraction (muscle tone). Loss of tone suggests interruption of nerve impulses.
Note

SKIN The skin is a durable, supple, waterproof membrane covering the entire body surface that protects against parasites, bacteria, viruses, and infection, holds body tissues and fluids, regulates body heat, and contains sensory nerves.
Definition and Function

Epidermis (*Outer Layer*)
Nonvascular dead cells
Pores
Pigment granules
Hair
Nails

Dermis (*Inner Layer*)
Blood vessels
Pore endings
Nerve endings
Hair and hair follicles
Glands: oil, sweat

Components

Skin color comes from blood circulating in subcutaneous (beneath the skin) vessels and pigment granules.
Note

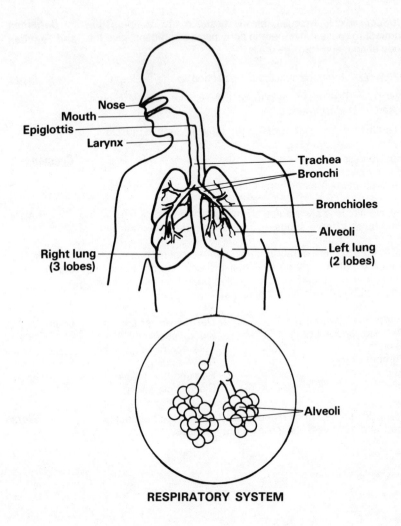

Nose
Mouth
Epiglottis
Larynx

Trachea
Bronchi

Bronchioles

Alveoli

Right lung
(3 lobes)

Left lung
(2 lobes)

Alveoli

RESPIRATORY SYSTEM

Respiratory System

The organs and structures of respiration that bring air into the lungs (inhalation) where O_2, CO_2, and waste products are exchanged, and return it to the atmosphere (exhalation)   ***Definition and Function***

Upper airway (passages above the larynx)   ***Components***
  Nose (nasal cavity)
  Mouth
  Pharynx (back of mouth)
  Epiglottis ("lid" over larynx)
Lower airway (passages below the larynx)
  Larynx (voice box)
  Trachea (windpipe)
  Bronchi (right and left branches)
  Lungs (left: two lobes; right: three lobes)
    Pleura (membrane covering the lung and lining the chest wall)
    Pleural space (space between two pleura)
    Bronchioles (air passages within the lungs)
    Alveoli (air sacs within the lungs)
Diaphragm (muscle/tissue partition separating thoracic and abdominal cavities)
Ribs and rib muscles

Normal respirations (per minute)   ***Normal Range***

Newborn,	30–50	6 years,	20–26
11 months,	26–40	8–10 years,	18–24
2–4 years,	20–30	Adolescent to adult,	12–20

Pain, fear, excitement, and anxiety also stimulate respiration.   ***Note***

Increased CO_2 in the blood stimulates breathing; decreased CO_2 depresses breathing.

Normal atmospheric air contains 21% O_2; exhaled air contains enough O_2 (16%) to support life.

The first priority in any emergency is to establish and maintain an adequate airway.   ***Remember***

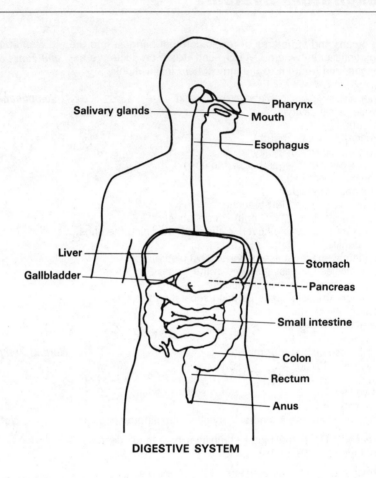

Salivary glands

Pharynx

Mouth

Esophagus

Liver

Gallbladder

Stomach

Pancreas

Small intestine

Colon

Rectum

Anus

DIGESTIVE SYSTEM

Digestive System

The organs, structures, and glands of the alimentary canal (digestive tube) that enable eating, digesting, and absorption of foods, and elimination of solid wastes   **Definition and Function**

Mouth   **Components**
  Salivary glands
  Pharynx (back of mouth)
Esophagus
Gastrointestinal tract
  Stomach
  Small intestine
  Large intestine
  Rectum
  Anus
Liver
Gallbladder
Pancreas

Muscular contractions (peristalsis) moving food and gas   **Note**
through the intestines produce the bowel sounds heard when
auscultating (listening with stethoscope) the abdomen.

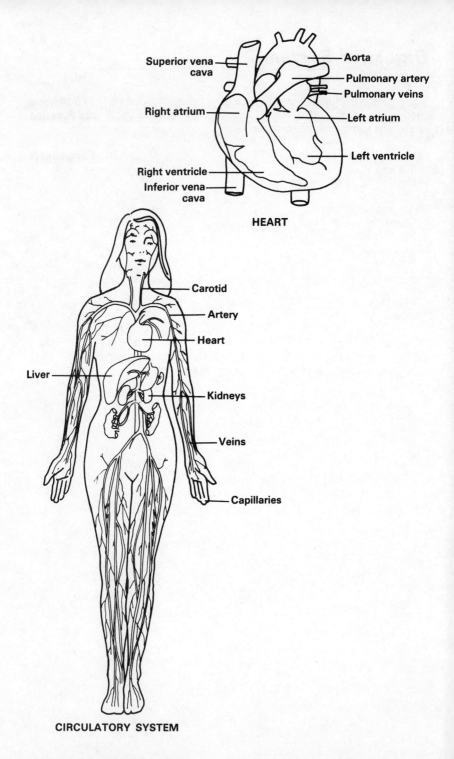

Superior vena cava

Aorta

Pulmonary artery

Pulmonary veins

Right atrium

Left atrium

Left ventricle

Right ventricle

Inferior vena cava

HEART

Carotid

Artery

Heart

Liver

Kidneys

Veins

Capillaries

CIRCULATORY SYSTEM

Circulatory System

A closed system of tubes through which blood carrying O_2, nutrients, CO_2, and wastes is circulated throughout the body under pressure generated by the heart to perfuse all living cells — ***Definition and Function***

Heart (four chambers) — ***Components***
   Right atrium (receives venous blood from body)
   Right ventricle (pumps venous blood to lungs)
   Left atrium (receives oxygenated blood from lungs)
   Left ventricle (pumps oxygenated blood to cells)
Veins (carry deoxygenated blood at low pressure)
Arteries (carry oxygenated blood at high pressure)
Capillaries (exchange O_2, CO_2, nutrients, and wastes)
Blood
   Plasma (fluid portion)
   Red blood cells (carry O_2)
   White blood cells (fight infection)
   Platelets (promote clotting)
Lymphatic system (returns tissue fluid to blood)

Arterial blood: bright red, pulsing flow — ***Note***
Venous blood: dark, blue-red, steady flow

Control of major bleeding is the third step of a primary survey (airway, breathing, circulation). — ***Remember***

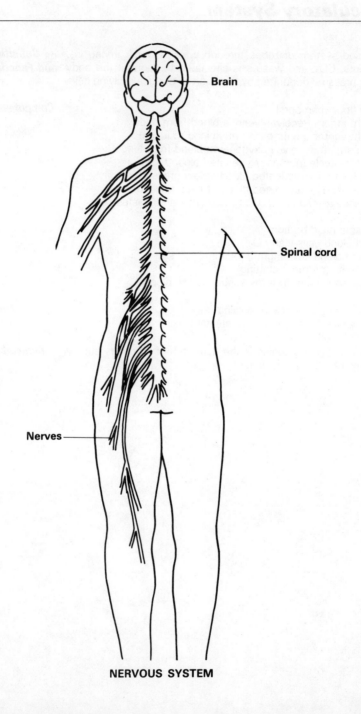

Brain

Spinal cord

Nerves

NERVOUS SYSTEM

Nervous System

The complex network of structures that activates, coordinates, and controls all body functions including sensation, movement, memory, and thought

Central nervous system
    Brain (master organ; encased by skull)
    Spinal cord (relay between nerves and brain; encased by
      spine)
Peripheral nervous system
    Nerves
        Sensory (carry sensations to brain)
        Motor (carry stimulus to muscles)
    Voluntary nervous system (regulates voluntary functions,
      e.g., walking, chewing, eye movement)
    Involuntary (autonomic) nervous system (regulates involun-
      tary functions, *e.g.*, heartbeat, digestion)

Components

Cerebrospinal fluid and three layers of protective membrane (meninges) surround the brain and spinal cord.

Presence of cerebrospinal fluid draining from a head wound, the ears, or the nose may indicate a skull fracture.

Note

Permanent paralysis or loss of function may result from brain, spinal cord, or nerve injury.

Remember

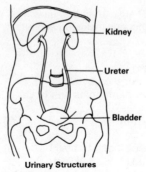

Urinary Structures

GENITOURINARY SYSTEM

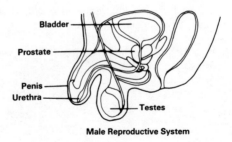

Male Reproductive System

Female Reproductive System

Genitourinary System

Two separate systems: the urinary system, the organs and structures that filter and excrete wastes from the blood; and the reproductive system, the organs and structures of reproduction

Definition and Function

Urinary System
Kidneys (2)
Ureters (2)
Bladder
Urethra

Components

Reproductive Systems
Male
  Testes (located in scrotum)
  Penis (contains urethra)
  Accessory
    Vas deferens, seminal vesicle, prostate
Female
  Ovaries
  Fallopian tubes
  Uterus
  Cervix
  Accessory
    Vagina, vulva, mammary glands

SECTION 2

Patient Assessment

This section reviews call and patient assessment procedures, the vital signs and their ranges, the order of treatment, multiple casualty classification principles, and shock.

Guidelines

1. The vital sign ranges are approximations, not absolutes.
2. Organization and order are essential to efficient patient assessment.
3. Thorough field assessments and surveys should include all the steps included in this section.
4. Personal preference and local protocol may determine the sequence of your surveys. Once you have established a sequence, don't vary it.

This section will help you to

1. Assess a call
2. Perform a primary and secondary survey
3. Review vital signs and their ranges
4. Determine treatment and transport priorities
5. Classify multiple casualties
6. Assess and treat a patient for shock

Shock is a syndrome that may appear in any patient. Observing for its signs and symptoms should be a part of every patient survey.

Note

Special Considerations

Environmental Factors
    Topography, terrain
    Weather, temperature, precipitation, wind chill
    Time of day (daylight, darkness)
    Routes, roads, access to scene, nearest medical facility
    Traffic
    Crowds
    Hazards: flood, fire, downed power lines
Support Services
    Police, fire department
    Civil defense, rescue groups
    Others (see p. 275)
Communications
    Mobile radio (ambulance)
    Portable radio (personal)
    Telephone
    Links to
        Hospital, EMS system
        Police department, fire department, rescue
        Mutual aid groups, personnel
Patient
    Age, weight, physical condition
    Handicap
    Pregnancy
    Medical history, chronic conditions, chief complaint, allergies
    Language spoken
    Attending physician
    Parents, guardian if minor or dependent
Patient Location (Scene)
    Access to scene: roads, driveways, stairways, halls
    Access to patient: stairs, halls, physical hazards, fire, smoke, chemicals, gas, crowds
    Crime scene

Call Assessment

1. *Assess incident* (What happened?) from
   a. Dispatcher (en route)
   b. Police, witnesses, bystanders (at scene)
   c. Patient, family, friends (with patient)
2. *Determine mechanism of injury* (How did it happen?)
3. *Note hazardous conditions* (before entering scene)
   a. Correct as necessary before proceeding
4. *Find all victims*
   a. Triage (sort out)
5. *Establish communications links* (radio, telephone)
   a. Dispatch
   b. Emergency room
   c. Police, fire, civil defense, disaster
6. *Request assistance* as required
   a. Additional medical personnel and equipment
   b. Extrication
   c. Police, fire, civil defense, bystanders
7. *Assess patient* (see Patient Assessment, p. 33, 35, 37)
8. *Treat patient*
9. *Transport*

1. *Assess nature of call* per dispatch
2. *Locate patient*
3. *Assess scene* for
   a. Transport problems (stairs, halls, etc.)
   b. Number of patients
   c. Need for assistance
4. *Establish communications* (radio, telephone)
   a. Dispatch
   b. Emergency room
   c. Police, other
5. *Request assistance* as required
6. *Assess patient* (see Patient Assessment, p. 33, 35, 37)
7. *Treat patient*
8. *Transport*

Expect the worst and be prepared for it.   *Note*

Your first obligation is your own safety.   *Remember*

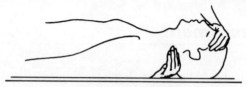

1. Open the airway

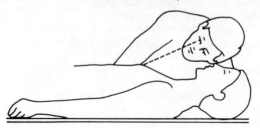

2. Check for breathing

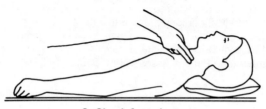

3. Check for pulse

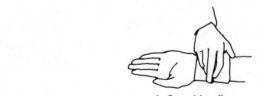

4. Stop bleeding

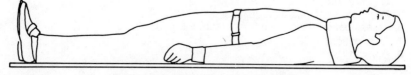

5. Check for spinal injuries; immobilize

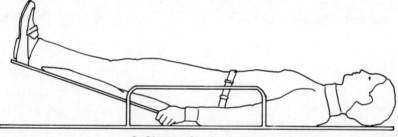

6. Observe for shock; treat

Primary Survey

The rapid detection and immediate correction of life-threatening conditions **Definition**

Airway   **Steps**
Look, listen, feel
Open, adequate, secure?
Correct at once
    Tilt head, lift chin, thrust jaw

Breathing
Adequate air exchange?
    a. Depth
    b. Difficulty (gasping, unusual patterns)
    c. Rate: *assist breathing* if under 10 per minute

Circulation
Pulse present? (carotid)
    a. *No Pulse: Initiate CPR at once*
    b. Rate
    c. Quality
    d. Regularity

Hemorrhage
External
    Stop severe bleeding at once: Direct pressure, pressure
        point, elevate, ice pack, tourniquet
Internal
    MAST (follow local protocol)
    Transport without delay

Spine
Is patient conscious? (see p. 47)
Is there evidence of CNS injury? (see p. 53)
*Stabilize neck and spine before moving whenever CNS injuries
    are suspected*

Shock
Are signs and symptoms of shock present? (see p. 61)
Stabilize and transport without delay

A primary survey must be done on every patient, in the same sequence, whether the patient is conscious or not.   **Note**

Treat all life-threatening conditions as they are found before proceeding with survey.   **Remember**

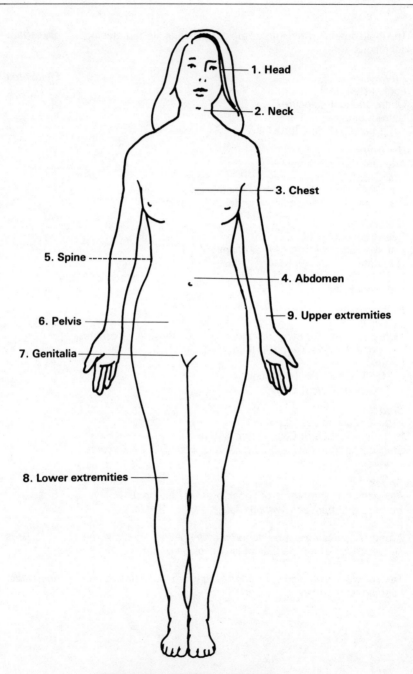

1. Head
2. Neck
3. Chest
5. Spine
4. Abdomen
9. Upper extremities
6. Pelvis
7. Genitalia
8. Lower extremities

SECONDARY SURVEY SEQUENCE

Secondary Survey

To locate problems that may develop into more serious or life-threatening conditions if not treated · **Definition**

Stethoscope, blood pressure cuff, watch (with second hand), penlight, heavy duty scissors, thermometer, survey form, pen · **Equipment Required**

Procedure

1. *Overall* condition and appearance
   a. Position found
   b. Level of consciousness
   c. General behavior, chief complaint, distress
   d. Obvious injuries, deformities
   e. Condition of skin
2. Head and neck
   a. Scalp (blood, lumps, cuts, depressions)
   b. Ears (trauma, blood, clear fluid)
   c. Eyes (trauma, swelling, ecchymosis, pupil equality, light reaction, sagging lids, redness, pus, blood in sclera or anterior chamber, foreign bodies, abnormal movement)
   d. Nose (trauma, blood, clear fluid, nasal flaring, deformity)
   e. Mouth (trauma, blood, vomitus, drooling, foreign material, dentures, odor)
   f. Lips (trauma, cyanosis, dry)
   g. Jaw (trauma, stability, crepitus)
   h. Skin (trauma, moisture, color, sagging, temperature)
   i. Neck (trauma, distended veins, deviated trachea, muscle spasm, stoma, Medic-alert tag, cervical spine irregularities)
3. Chest (flail chest, diaphragmatic breathing, malformations, intercostal retractions, tenderness, trauma, breath sounds)
4. Abdomen (trauma, distention, lumps, discoloration, hardness, tenderness)
5. Spine (deformity, tenderness, muscle spasm)
6. Pelvis/genitalia (trauma, pain, tenderness, crepitus, priapism, incontinence)
7. Lower extremities (trauma, angulation, range and equality of movement, sensation, edema, pulses)
8. Upper extremities (trauma, angulation, range and equality of movement, sensation, pulses, nailbeds)

Include vital signs with survey. · **Note**

Effective Communicating

1. Introduce yourself and explain who you are
2. Explain what you are doing and what you are going to do
3. Let the patient speak and ask questions
4. Answer the patient's questions in understandable terms
5. Allow the patient to express feelings (guilt, fear, anxiety)
6. Help the patient to deal with his feelings
7. Be sympathetic and nonjudgmental
8. Don't patronize the patient or trivialize his condition and concern
9. Maintain a calm, assured, caring attitude
10. Listen carefully to the patient, family, witnesses
11. Provide emotional support
12. Inspire confidence by displaying professional skill, knowledge, and behavior

Patient History

Information obtained from the patient and others about the patient's condition to facilitate making an effective emergency care plan

PATIENT INTERVIEW

A. Determine the chief complaint
  a. *What* is the problem?
  b. *Where* is the problem?
  c. *When* did it start?
  d. *Why* did it start?
B. Determine its characteristics
  a. *Quality* (Describe the pain.)
  b. *Intensity* (How bad is the pain?)
  c. *Frequency* (How often does it hurt?)
  d. *Aggravation* (What makes it feel worse?)
  e. *Relief* (What makes it feel better?)
C. Determine associated complaints
  a. *What else* is wrong?

MEDICAL HISTORY
A. Interview the patient, relatives, and friends
  a. What other medical problems are being treated?
  b. What medications are being taken?
  c. What allergies does the patient have?
  d. Has the patient had treatment or hospitalization for recent injury or illness? What? When? Where?
  e. Who is the patient's physician?
  f. Obtain pertinent family history

Don't assume that a patient who can't or doesn't speak can't understand.

Avoid asking questions that can be answered with a "yes" or "no."

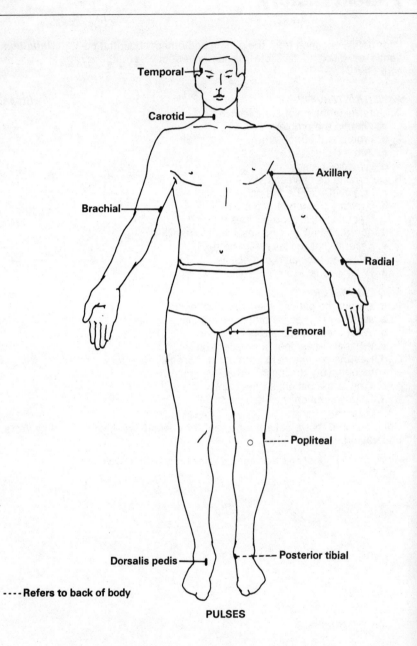

Temporal

Carotid

Axillary

Brachial

Radial

Femoral

Popliteal

Dorsalis pedis

Posterior tibial

----Refers to back of body

PULSES

The rhythmic movement of blood through arteries that corresponds to the heartbeat and can be felt when an artery near the body surface is palpated   ***Definition***

Watch with second hand, stethoscope*   ***Equipment***

Place finger(s) only over pulse location, count pulses in 30 seconds, multiply by 2 for heartbeats per minute. If irregular, count for a full minute.   ***Method***

(*Alternative method: listen at apex of heart, approximately 2 in below left nipple with stethoscope for apical beat.)

Temporal: at base of temple, anterior to ear   ***Locations***
Carotid: in groove alongside trachea
Axillary: in middle of armpit
Brachial: 1 in above elbow crease, slightly medial
Radial: at wrist, proximal to base of thumb
Femoral: in groin medial to junction of trunk and hip
Popliteal: medial to space behind knee
Posterior tibial: posterior to medial malleolus
Dorsalis pedis: on foot lateral to big toe tendon

Heartbeats (pulse) per minute   ***Normal***
Newborn, 70–170 (average, 120)   6 years,   75–115   ***Ranges***
11 months, 80–160   8–10 years, 70–110
 2 years   80–130   Adolescent, 60–110
 4 years, 80–120   Adult,   60–80

Rate: number of beats per minute   ***Evaluation***
Rhythm: regular; irregular
Strength: strong; weak; thready

The most reliable pulses are (1) carotid and (2) femoral.   ***Note***

The radial pulse is most commonly used during the secondary survey.

Pulse rate varies with age, sex, physical condition, amount of exercise, medications, blood loss, stress, fear, and anxiety.

Do not take both carotid pulses simultaneously.   ***Caution***

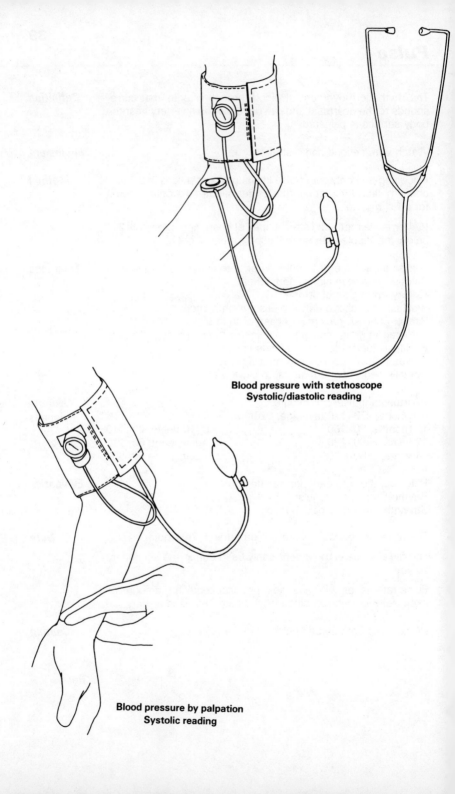

**Blood pressure with stethoscope
Systolic/diastolic reading**

**Blood pressure by palpation
Systolic reading**

Blood Pressure

The pressure of circulating blood against arterial walls | *Definition*

Blood pressure cuff, stethoscope | *Equipment*

Place cuff 1 in above left elbow crease with "Artery" arrow | *Method*
over brachial artery; with stethoscope diaphragm over brachial
artery, inflate cuff to between 180 and 220 mmHg; deflate
slowly; record systolic/diastolic pressures.

		Normal Ranges
Male		
Systolic	100 + age to 150 (95–140)	
Diastolic	66–90 (60–90)	
Female	8–10 less than for male	
Newborn (average)	74/40	
To 1 year	85/60	
2–6 years	90/60	
6–10 years	95/62	
10–18 years	105/65	

PALPATION | *Variations*
Apply cuff and stethoscope as above; on same arm, locate
radial artery with finger; inflate cuff 20 mmHg past point at
which radial pulse disappears; deflate slowly; point at which
pulse returns is systolic pressure.

PALPATED PULSES
If pulses are palpable, systolic BP is

Radial, 80
Brachial, 70
Femoral, 60
Carotid, 50

(Readings are usually 10 mmHg below stethoscope readings.)

Wrong cuff size: if too small, false high reading, if too large, | *Errors*
false low reading; hearing sounds incorrectly; wrong placement
of cuff over artery; cuff too loose.

Posture changes vary readings; wait and repeat. | *Note*

Blood pressure alone is not the sole indicator of the severity or | *Caution*
urgency of a patient's condition.

Pain, anxiety, medical condition, drugs, and activity affect blood | *Remember*
pressure.

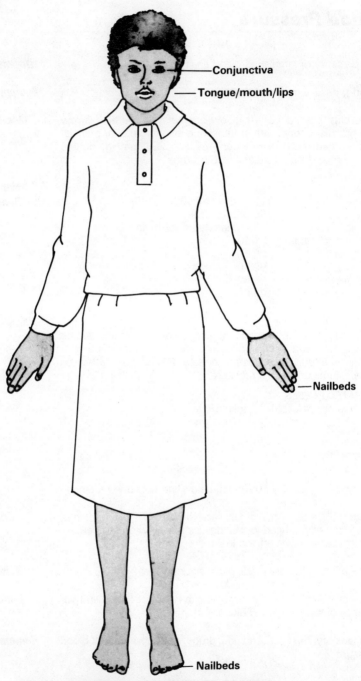

Conjunctiva

Tongue/mouth/lips

Nailbeds

Nailbeds

COLOR CHANGES IN DARK-SKINNED PATIENT

Skin Color

An indication of the presence of circulating blood and O_2 in subcutaneous tissues, and of certain diseases* **Definition**

Face, lips, nailbeds, mouth (mucous membranes), earlobes, eyes (conjunctiva) **Location**

Color	Indicates	Variations
Red	Alcohol ingestion, diabetic coma, allergic reaction, cold weather, heart attack, rising BP, blushing, CVA	
Red, hot	Infection, external heat, sunburn, burn, heat stroke	
Cherry red	CO poisoning, heat stroke	
White, pale/cool	Fear, hypovolemia, heat exhaustion, poor circulation, shock, fainting, emotional stress, shock, blood loss	
White, moist	Heart attack	
White, dry	Hypothermia, anemia	
Blue	Cyanosis, hypovolemia, CHF, airway obstruction, embolism, pulmonary edema, cold weather, asphyxia, heart attack	
*Yellow	Liver disease, gallbladder inflammation, jaundice, hepatitis, uremic disorder	
Mottled white/blue	Cardiac arrest	
Bruise, black/blue	Blunt force injury (may take 24–48 hours to appear)	
Bruise, yellow	Old bruise	
Hematoma	Rapid pooling of subcutaneous blood; indicates large vessel injury	

On a dark-skinned patient, look for color changes in nailbeds, under tongue, in eyes (conjunctiva). Signs of shock: gray cast around nose and mouth; mouth, tongue, lips, and nailbeds are blue. **Attention**

Assess skin color of every patient. **Note**

44

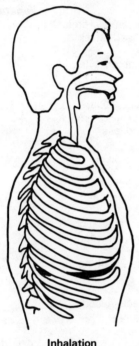

**Inhalation
(Lungs inflate)**

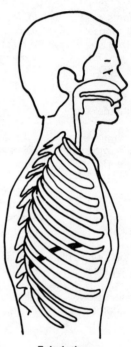

**Exhalation
(Lungs deflate)**

Respiration (*Breathing*)

Taking air into the lungs (inhalation) and expelling it to the atmo-sphere (exhalation)
Definition

Watch with second hand; stethoscope
Equipment

LOOK Observe and count chest rise and fall (number of breaths per minute = rate), watch movement of diaphragm, look for nostril flaring, look for intercostal soft tissue and muscle bulging and retraction
Method

LISTEN Listen at nose and mouth with ear; listen to chest with stethoscope

FEEL Feel the patient's chest rise and diaphragm movement with your hands.

Respiration rate per minute
Infant, 20–30
Child, 18–26
Adult, 12–20
Normal Ranges

Rate	Breaths per minute	*Evaluate*
Rhythm	Slow, rapid, irregular	
Depth	Deep, shallow	
Ease	Easy, labored, painful	
Odor	Alcohol, acetone (fruity), chemicals	
Sounds	Stridor (crowing), wheezes (high-pitched), rales (fine crackling), rhonchi (louder, coarser, wet-ter than rales), gurgling	
Movement	Chest (paradoxical, asymmetrical), accessory muscle (diaphragm/upper abdomen)	

Cheyne-Stokes respiration (abnormal): a repeating 45 seconds to 3 minutes cycle of slow/shallow–deep/rapid–slow/shallow–apnea (no breathing); associated with head trauma and with metabolic and neurologic conditions.
Note

Hypopnea: fewer than 10 respirations/minute

Tachypnea: more than 30 respirations/minute

How to Score Responses to the Glasgow Coma Scale

Scoring of Eye Opening: 4 if the patient opens his eyes spontaneously; 3 if the patient opens his eyes in response to speech (spoken or shouted); 2 if the patient opens his eyes only in response to painful stimuli such as digital squeezing around nailbeds; 1 if the patient does not open his eyes in response to painful stimuli.

Scoring of Best Motor Response: 6 if the patient can obey a simple command such as "Lift your left hand off the bed"; 5 if the patient moves a limb to locate the painful stimuli applied to the head or trunk and attempts to remove the source; 4 if the patient attempts to withdraw from the source of pain; 3 if the patient flexes only his arms at the elbows and wrist in response to painful stimuli to the nailbeds (decorticate rigidity); 2 if the patient extends his arms (straightens his elbows) in response to painful stimuli (decerebrate rigidity); 1 if the patient has no motor response to pain on any limb.

Scoring of Best Verbal Response: 5 if the patient is oriented to time, place, and person; 4 if the patient is able to converse although not oriented to time, place, or person (*e.g.*, "Where am I?"); 3 if the patient speaks only in words or phrases that make little or no sense; 2 if the patient responds with incomprehensible sounds such as groans; 1 if the patient does not respond verbally at all.

(Hickey, JV: Clinical Practice of Neurological and Neurosurgical Nursing, 2nd ed. Philadelphia, JB Lippincott, 1986)

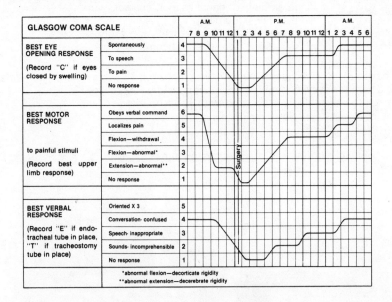

Level of Consciousness

The degree of awareness of one's surroundings | ***Definition***

Alert: Awake; appropriate auditory, visual, and tactile responses; correctly oriented to person (Who am I?), place (Where am I?), and time (What day is it?) | ***States***
Lethargic: Will fall asleep if undisturbed, but is easily awakened by voice or touch
Stuporous: Lethargic and unaware of surroundings; can be awakened by loud noise or vigorous shaking, but falls asleep rapidly
Delirious: Confused, disoriented, restless, incoherent, frightened, anxious
Coma: Profoundly unconscious, cannot be awakened

Evaluate the following: | ***Assessment***
Orientation: Is patient alert?
Verbal response: Are answers and actions appropriate, assured, and timely?
Activity: Is patient active, movement meaningful?
Motor response: Does patient respond to pain (pin-prick, squeeze, pressure) equally on both sides of body?

The level of consciousness is probably the best indicator of | ***Note***
nervous system condition. Note all changes; rapid deterioration indicates the need for urgent medical attention.

Corneal reflex (eye closing on touch to cornea) and gag reflex are last to disappear.

Don't confuse fear, CVA signs and symptoms, mental illness, or language barrier with deteriorating level of consciousness.

Refer to Glasgow Coma Scale, facing page.

Conditions Causing Increase or Absence of Pain

Shock; spinal cord damage; alcohol and drug abuse; circulatory impairment; medication; psychological reactions; anxiety; fear; previous injury at same location; previous similar attack; medical or physical condition

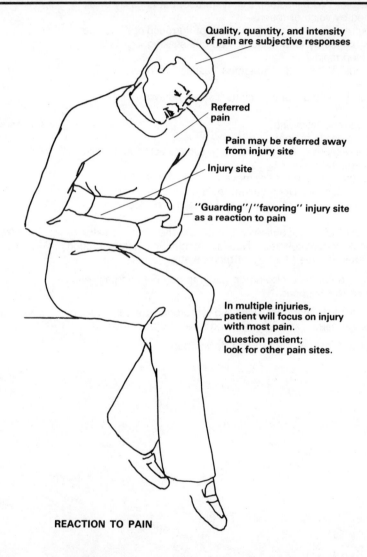

Quality, quantity, and intensity of pain are subjective responses

Referred pain

Pain may be referred away from injury site

Injury site

"Guarding"/"favoring" injury site as a reaction to pain

In multiple injuries, patient will focus on injury with most pain.

Question patient; look for other pain sites.

REACTION TO PAIN

Reaction to Pain

A response to unpleasant sensations caused by noxious stimuli **Definition**

Autonomic: changes in involuntary vital functions (heart, **Types of**
  smooth muscle, glands) **Reactions**
Skeletal muscle: loss of voluntary movement, "guarding" or
  "favoring" injured part
Psychic: patient's response; how patient deals with pain

Obtain patient's responses to the following questions: **History**
Location   Where is it?
Quality   What is it like?
Intensity   How bad is it?
Quantity   How much is there?
Chronology   When did it start?
Frequency   How often does it appear?
Setting   What makes it begin?
Aggravation   What makes it worse?
Alleviation   What makes it better?
Other pain   What else hurts?

Mild; moderate; severe; chronic; acute; burning; sharp; dull; **Description**
diffuse; referred

1. Accept patient's perception and description of the pain **Management**
2. Discuss with patient
   a. How it affects activities
   b. How it was managed before
   c. How it can be relieved
3. Tell patient how and when relief can be expected
4. Use pain relief techniques (splinting, elevation, positioning,
   pillows, O_2, relaxation)

Pain is a warning of something wrong. Locating it usually points **Note**
to the cause of a patient's problem; however, lack of pain does
not mean there is no problem.

Quality, intensity, and quantity are subjective responses influ-
enced by childhood pain experiences.

Pain in children is often global rather than local.

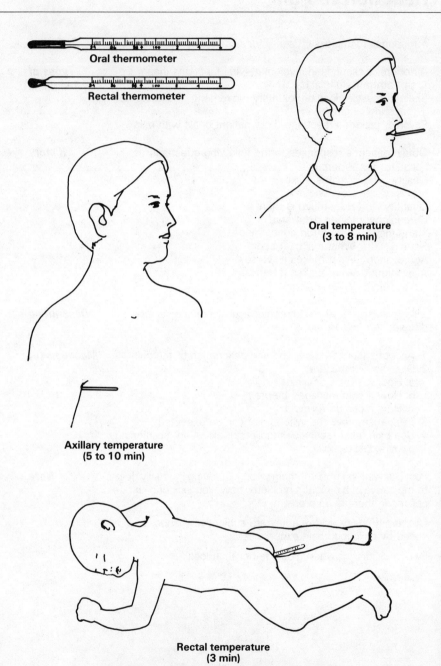

Oral thermometer

Rectal thermometer

**Oral temperature
(3 to 8 min)**

**Axillary temperature
(5 to 10 min)**

**Rectal temperature
(3 min)**

Immobilize infant and thermometer during procedure

Temperature

The relative measure of body heat	*Definition*

Thermometer (oral, rectal, disposable, electronic)	*Equipment*

Oral	97.6°F–99°F (average, 98.6°F)	*Normal Range*
Rectal	98.6°F–100°F	
Axillary	96.6°F–98°F	

Oral	Oral thermometer placed under tongue with mouth closed for 3–8 minutes	*Method*
Rectal	Lubricated rectal thermometer inserted 1 inch into rectum for minimum of 3 minutes (most accurate measure)	
Axillary	Thermometer held in bare armpit for 5–10 minutes (least accurate)	
Touch	Place back of hand against patient's skin (forehead, cheek, back of neck); gives relative temperature only	

Cool, moist (clammy)	Shock, bleeding, heat exhaustion	*Evaluation*
Cool, dry	Cold exposure, hypothermia	
Hot, dry	Fever, heat stroke, infection	
Hot, moist	Infection, external heat	
Fever	Warm, flushed skin, tachycardia, chills, night sweats	

Temperature differences in an extremity or between paired extremities may indicate impaired circulation.   *Note*

A hot region may indicate infection or inflammation.

Patients with high temperatures are more comfortable in a warm room, wearing few clothes so heat can dissipate.

Shivering and goosebumps are associated with heat loss, fear, pain, and disease.

Loss of Sensation (*Pain, Temperature, Touch, Pressure*)

Area of Injury	*Region of Sensory Loss*
C1–C4	Neck and below
C5–C7	Arms, hands, chest, abdomen, lower extremities
T1–T6	Mid-chest and below
T7–T12	Waist and below
L1–L3	Lower abdomen, legs
L4–L5	Parts of lower legs, feet
S1–S5	Posterior medial thigh, perineum, lateral foot

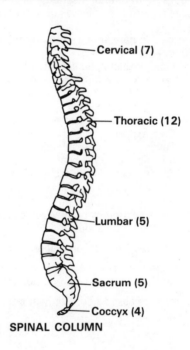

Cervical (7)

Thoracic (12)

Lumbar (5)

Sacrum (5)

Coccyx (4)

SPINAL COLUMN

Paralysis

The reduction or loss of voluntary movement   *Definition*

		Types
Quadriplegia	Paralysis of both arms and both legs	
Hemiplegia	Paralysis of arm and leg on one side	
Paraplegia	Paralysis of both legs	

Examine spine from top to bottom for deformity, blood, point   *Evaluation*
tenderness, protrusion, muscle spasm, and swelling.

Note voluntary movement, sensation, and reaction to pain from
head to toe; have patient do the following:
Face: open his eyes wide and close; wrinkle his forehead;
  show his teeth; and stick out his tongue
Arms/hands: raise his arm; squeeze your hand; move his
  fingers; feel your touch
Legs/feet: move his leg; press his foot against your hand;
  wiggle his toes; feel your touch

Suspect total or partial paralysis when   *Assessment*
1. Patient cannot move arms or legs
2. Muscles sag (face, extremities)
3. Muscles are weak, tender, or in spasm
4. Movements lack coordination
5. Signs and symptoms of CVA are present (see p. 205)
6. Patient breathes diaphragmatically
7. Mechanism of injury involves flexion, extension, or rotation
   of neck or head
8. Consciousness impaired, neurogenic shock

A patient with a severed spinal cord is immediately and perma-   *Note*
nently paralyzed below the level of injury.

A gradually compressing spinal injury produces a gradual pro-
gression of paralysis.

Any patient complaining of numbness or tingling in the extremi-   *Remember*
ties should be treated and immobilized as a spinal injury.

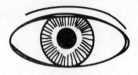 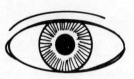

Normal

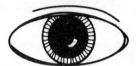 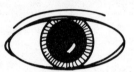

Dilated

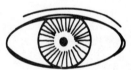 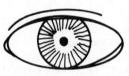

Constricted

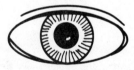 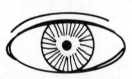

Unequal

PUPILS

Pupils

Circular (black) opening in the center of iris that opens and closes in response to light, emotions, and certain drugs and medications
Definition

Light source (penlight, flashlight, daylight)
Equipment

Briefly direct light at one eye, and observe for pupil contraction and ability of eye to follow light. Remove light, and observe for dilation. Repeat with the opposite eye, and compare the responses.
Procedure

PERLA—Pupils Equal Reactive Light and Accommodation (Pupils are the same size, follow movement, and adjust to changes in light.)
Normal

Abnormal

Finding	Suspect
Dilated	Shock, unconsciousness, cardiac arrest, head/brain/CNS injury, drug use, blindness, fear, hypoxia, pain
Constricted	Head/brain/CNS injury, drug use, poisoning, bright light, old age
Unequal	Head injury, CVA, postcataract surgery, normal (2%–4% of population)
No response	Coma, death, cataract, false eye
Pinpoint (unreactive)	CNS damage, drug use
Lackluster (unreactive)	Coma, shock
Fixed or restricted gaze	Eye orbit fracture

Unequal pupil size in an injured patient is a reliable sign of head injury.
Note

Change in pupil size from dilated to more normal during CPR may indicate that brain is getting O_2.

Accurate pupil assessment is difficult in patients with contact lenses, artificial eye or lens, cataracts, or cataract surgery.
Remember

First Priority

Airway and breathing problems
Cardiac arrest
Uncontrolled or suspected severe bleeding
Severe head trauma
Severe medical emergency
   Poisoning
   Diabetic emergency
   Cardiac emergency
Open chest and abdominal wounds
Shock

Second Priority

Burns
Major or multiple fractures
Back, neck, and spine injuries

Third Priority

Uncomplicated fractures
Minor injuries
Mortal injury, death imminent
Dead
Cardiac arrest without enough personnel to care for numerous other
patients

Note   Follow local protocol.

Priorities

The order of treatment and transport determined by the severity of a patient's condition — *Definition*

FIRST PRIORITY (1, HIGH, EMERGENT) — *Levels*
Life- or function-threatening conditions requiring immediate medical attention
Treat and transport immediately

SECOND PRIORITY (2, MEDIUM, URGENT)
Potentially dangerous conditions if untreated within a few hours
Treat and Transport without delay

THIRD PRIORITY (3, LOW, NONEMERGENT)
Conditions that require routine or no immediate medical attention
Treat and transport last

1. Primary survey (ABC) — *Assessment*
Yields first priority, or proceed to
2. Secondary survey (head to toe)
Yields first, second, and third priorities, then
3. Monitor patient for changes in
  a. Breathing
  b. Level of consciousness
  c. Vital signs
4. Change priority as indicated by status change

Increasing respiratory distress; progressive shock; falling pulse pressure (difference between systolic and diastolic reading); rapidly deteriorating level of consciousness; coma following a lucid period; airway and chest wall problems; sudden hypotension with possible GI bleeding; penetrating wounds of head, chest, and abdomen — *Special Attention*

Designate team leader or most qualified medically trained person on team to determine priorities. — *Note*

Priorities reflect a condition's severity of danger to the patient, not the patient's or the injury's appearance.

58

Evacuation Priorities

1. Patients in danger of death from bleeding, asphyxia, severe thoracic injuries, or shock
2. Stabilized patients in danger of shock; patients with closed head injuries and decreasing level of consciousness
3. Spinal cord, eye, hand, and large muscle area injuries; major compound fractures
4. Soft tissue injuries; uncomplicated fractures
5. Ambulatory injured patients

Special Attention Situations

1. High-speed (35 MPH and higher) motor vehicle accident
2. Rapid deceleration and acceleration; abrupt forces
3. Unconsciousness following injury
4. Inappropriate behavior suggesting head injury (denies obvious injury; abnormal speech or thought)
5. Chest and abdominal pain following injury
6. Multiple rib fractures
7. Danger of aspiration
8. Danger of lung tissue injury
9. Pulse over 100 (patient at rest)
10. Head *and* cervical spine injury
11. Falls higher than 15 feet
12. Patients under the influence of drugs or alcohol
13. Patients with a history of severe medical diseases

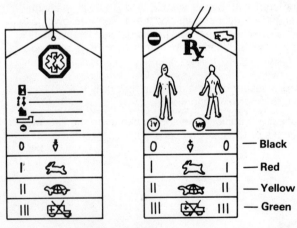

- Black
- Red
- Yellow
- Green

TRIAGE TAGS

Triage

The classification of multiple casualties based on the gravity of injuries or illness and the urgency of treatment and transport **Definition**

MULTIPLE PATIENT **Types**
An emergency incident with more than one patient that is manageable by one or more responding units without declaring a mass casualty disaster.

MASS CASUALTY DISASTER
A multiple patient emergency incident that requires implementation of an EMS disaster plan.

To select the order of patient treatment based on **Principle**
1. Death is imminent (within minutes)
2. Death is likely (within hours)
3. No serious injuries, or death has occurred

First (red tag); second (yellow tag); third (green tag) **Priorities**

Triage leader (EMT in charge, or most medically qualified) does **Guidelines** primary survey only, evaluates priorities for treatment and transport, and determines what other help (EMS, fire, police, rescue personnel) is needed at scene.

Routine triage team responsibilities: prevent further injury, accident, and damage; sort and protect patients; direct bystanders; reassure survivors and relatives.

Do not assume the roles of police or other authorities when that authority is represented at the scene.

In a disaster, it is better to request too much help than not **Note** enough.

Care is concentrated on those likely to survive.

Saving a life precedes saving a limb.

Assume the worst and be prepared to deal with it.

Types of Shock

Anaphylactic	Severe allergic reaction
Cardiogenic	Low cardiac output
Hypovolemic	Blood loss, inadequate blood volume
Metabolic	Blood chemistry imbalance
Neurogenic	Blood vessel nerve control loss
Psychogenic	Temporary vessel dilation due to fear
Respiratory	Inadequate or inefficient respirations
Septic	Severe infection

Causes of Shock

Blood loss	Emotional stress	Electric shock
Severe pain	Allergic reactions	Extreme heat or cold
Severe injury	Severe burns	Toxic poisoning

Shock Thresholds

Shock is indicated when systolic BP is below

90	Adult male	60	Pre-teens (5–12 years)
80	Adult female	50	Child under 5 years
70	Young adult or teenager		

Anaphylactic Shock (a True Emergency)

Signs and symptoms
1. Itching, burning, flushed skin (chest and face)
2. Hives; swollen face, tongue; cyanosis (lips)
3. Tightness, pain in chest; respiratory distress, wheezing
4. Weak pulse
5. Dizziness, faintness, coma

Treatment
1. See Treatment, facing page
2. Assist patient self administer medication (follow local protocol)
3. Transport *at once*

Shock Prevention

1. Control bleeding
2. Secure and maintain airway
3. Loosen tight clothing
4. Immobilize fractures
5. Relieve pain
6. Reassure patient

Note

SHOCK SIGNS IN DARK-SKINNED PATIENTS
Gray skin around nose and mouth
Blue (cyanosis)—lips, tongue, mouth, nailbeds

FACTORS AFFECTING DEGREE OF SHOCK
Pain; age, health, physical and medical condition; fatigue; incorrect assessment and care at scene

Shock

1 *Priority*

A syndrome (group of signs and symptoms) signalling the body's reaction to physical or emotional injury, caused by a decrease in the effective circulating blood volume due to blood loss or peripheral vascular collapse and the body's attempts to compensate *Definition*

1. Weakness, restlessness, anxiety, dizziness
2. Extreme thirst
3. Nausea, vomiting
4. Pale, cold, clammy skin; profuse sweating
5. Weak, thready, rapid (tachycardia) pulse
6. Shallow, rapid (tachypnea) breathing
7. Dilated pupils, lackluster eyes, lids droop or close
8. Falling or unobtainable blood pressure
9. Changing level of consciousness (confusion, coma)
10. Cyanosis: lips, earlobes, skin (later sign)
11. Fear; feeling of impending doom

Signs and Symptoms

1. Lay the patient down
2. Establish and maintain airway
3. Stop serious bleeding
4. Administer O_2 (high concentration; nonrebreather)
5. Elevate legs 8–12 in
6. Keep patient warm (cover with a blanket)
7. Immobilize fractures
8. Monitor level of consciousness and vital signs
9. Watch for respiratory distress, nausea, vomiting
10. Handle patient gently
11. Give nothing by mouth
12. Apply MAST if indicated (follow local protocol)

Treatment

Do not elevate legs when patient has head or chest injuries; raise upper body slightly; when in doubt, lay flat. *Caution*

Treat for shock before everything but breathing and bleeding emergencies. *Note*

Treat for shock *before* blood pressure drops.

The period before the point of irreversible shock decreases with severity of cause; treat before that point.

SECTION 3

This section reviews airway maintenance, cardiopulmonary resuscitation (CPR), and oxygen therapy, including mechanical aids and equipment.

Guidelines

1. When breathing stops, the heart stops and the patient is *clinically dead.*
2. If respiration resumes within 4 to 6 minutes, little or no tissue death occurs and recovery may be unaffected.
3. Irreversible brain damage occurs after 4 to 6 minutes of oxygen deprivation, followed quickly by *biological death.*
4. Artificial ventilation and CPR may prevent or minimize tissue damage from oxygen deprivation, and may prevent biological death.
5. Artificial ventilation is reviewed on page 66.
6. The CPR review sequences conform to standard procedures.

This section will help you to

1. Support patient breathing
2. Provide artificial ventilation and CPR
3. Review breathing aids
4. Administer oxygen

Always follow local protocol when assisting breathing, performing CPR, using mechanical aids, or administering oxygen.

Note

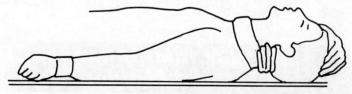

Open airway

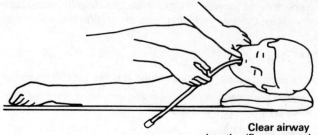

**Clear airway
(suction/fingersweep)**

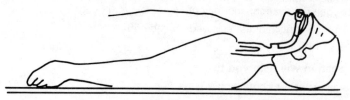

**Adjunct airway
(oropharyngeal airway)**

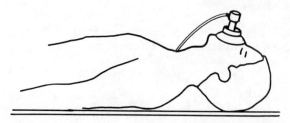

**Artificial ventilation
(demand valve)**

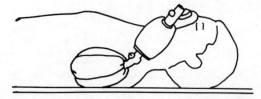

**Assist ventilation
(bag valve mask)**

Airway Maintenance

Establishment and support of a patent (open and unobstructed) airway **Definition**

Ineffective Airway **Signs and**
Abnormal breath sounds (crowing, wheezing, gurgling) **Symptoms**
Apnea (no breathing)
Changes in respiration rate or depth
Choking
Coughing
Cyanosis
Dyspnea (shortness of breath; difficulty breathing)
Inability to speak or cough

Procedures used (one, some, all, none) are determined by the **Procedures**
patient's condition.
1. Open airway (head tilt, chin lift, jaw thrust)
2. Clear airway (suction, fingersweep)
3. Artificial ventilation
4. Adjunct airway (oropharyngeal, nasopharyngeal, esophogeal
obturator airway [EOA])
5. Assist ventilations with 100% oxygen

The first step in opening the airway is to protect the cervical **Caution**
spine.

Do not use adjunct airways in a patient whose gag reflex is
intact.

Place unconscious patient in coma position; watch for vomiting; prepare to suction.

Do not suction longer than 5 to 10 seconds at one time.

Causes of Airway Obstruction

Tongue	Laryngospasm	Pneumothorax
Bronchospasm	COPD	Foreign object
Choking	Goiter	Mucus
Croup	Tumor	Food

Artificial Ventilation

1. Determine unresponsiveness; call for help
2. Open patient's airway
   a. Head tilt, neck lift
   b. Head tilt, chin lift
   c. Jaw thrust if neck injury suspected
3. Look, listen, and feel for breathing (3–5 seconds)
4. If no breathing, give two full slow breaths
5. Check for carotid pulse (5–10 seconds)
6. If pulse present, give one full slow breath every 5 seconds for 1 minute (12 breaths)
7. Reassess pulse, breathing
8. If no breathing, continue artificial ventilation

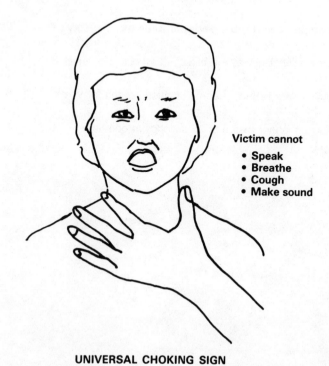

Victim cannot
- **Speak**
- **Breathe**
- **Cough**
- **Make sound**

UNIVERSAL CHOKING SIGN

Airway Obstruction: Adult

1   *Priority*

Partial or complete mechanical blockage of the airway   *Definition*

1. Patient can't speak, breathe, or make a sound   *Signs and*
2. Universal choking sign (patient clutches neck)   *Symptoms*
3. Cyanosis (face turns blue or gray color)
4. Desperate, ineffective breathing movements
5. Collapse, unconsciousness

CONSCIOUS PATIENT   *Procedure*
Partial obstruction
1. Do not interfere; encourage coughing

Complete obstruction
1. Ask, "Are you choking?"
2. Support patient upright, call for help
3. Deliver abdominal thrusts
4. Repeat until airway is cleared or patient becomes unconscious

UNCONSCIOUS PATIENT (obstructed)
1. Place patient supine; open airway
2. Ventilate mouth to mouth
3. Reposition airway if step 2 ineffective
4. Reattempt mouth-to-mouth ventilations
5. Deliver 6–10 abdominal thrusts (straddle patient)
6. Open mouth with tongue-jaw lift
7. Fingersweep mouth with face up
8. Reposition head and airway; ventilate
9. Repeat steps 5–7 until obstruction is cleared

Advanced pregnant patient: use chest thrusts only   *Variations*
Obese patient: use chest thrusts only

Patients in respiratory distress should receive O$_2$ immediately.   *Remember*

Do not exert pressure against patient's rib cage with forearms.   *Note*

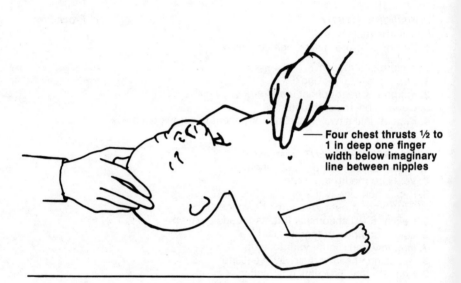

Four chest thrusts ½ to 1 in deep one finger width below imaginary line between nipples

Airway Obstruction

Airway Obstruction: Infant and Child

1   *Priority*

Partial or complete mechanical blockage of the airway in an   *Definition*
infant or child

1. Choking, gasping, unable to make a sound   *Signs and*
2. Cyanosis   *Symptoms*
3. Breathing stops
4. Universal choking sign (patient clutches neck)

CONSCIOUS PATIENT
1. If forceful coughing occurs, leave patient alone
2. If breathing is stopped or ineffective
   a. Call for help
   b. Give four back blows
   c. Give four chest thrusts (two–three fingers on sternum,
       one finger width below imaginary line between nipples)
       only on infants up to 1 year of age
3. Repeat steps **b** and **c** until obstruction is expelled or infant
   becomes unconscious

UNCONSCIOUS PATIENT
1. Call for help; activate EMS
2. Place patient supine
3. Deliver sequence **b** and **c** above
4. Tongue-jaw lift to visualize obstruction
   a. If visible, remove with fingers
   b. If not visible, do not attempt removal with fingers
5. Attempt to ventilate if obstruction not visible
6. Repeat steps 2 and 3, if airway is still blocked, until successful

Do not hang infant by his feet to dislodge foreign matter from   *Warning*
throat.

Chest thrusts are the same as CPR compressions.   *Note*

Forceful coughing means airway is partially open; *do not* inter- *Remember*
vene until it is completely obstructed.

Chances to clear obstructed airway improve as muscles relax;
continue efforts until successful.

Avoid blind fingersweeps.

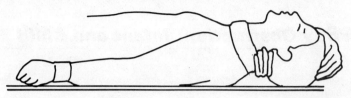

Open airway

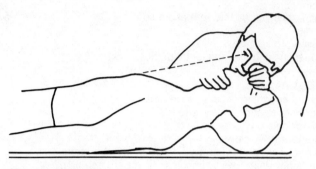

Give two slow full breaths (watch for chest rise)

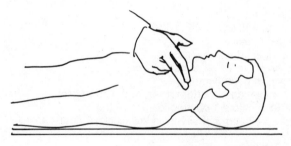

Check carotid pulse

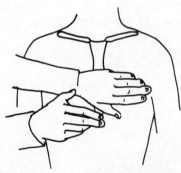

Hand placement for chest compressions

CPR *(Cardiopulmonary Resuscitation)*: **Adult**

Artificial ventilation with external cardiac massage (chest compressions) performed on patients in cardiac arrest

Definition

CARDIAC ARREST
1. Absence of pulse
2. Absence of breathing

Signs and Symptoms

ONE-RESCUER CPR
1. Recognize unconsciousness (shake patient and shout)
2. Summon help
3. Position patient (logroll if spine injury is suspected)
4. Open airway (tilt head or lift chin)
5. Look, listen, and feel for breathing (3 to 5 seconds)
6. Give two slow full breaths (watch for chest to rise)
7. Check carotid pulse (5 to 10 seconds)
8. If no pulse, give 15 compressions in 9–11 seconds, 1½–2 in deep, 80–100/s
9. Give two slow full breaths
10. Complete four cycles (15 : 2)
11. Check pulse and breathing
12. If absent, give two slow full breaths
13. Resume CPR until patient recovers, you are relieved or exhausted, or patient is pronounced dead

Procedure

ENTRY OF SECOND RESCUER
1. Steps 1–7 (above) until second rescuer arrives
2. First rescuer:"Take over compressions"
3. First rescuer reassesses pulse and breathing as second rescuer positions self to give compressions
4. If no pulse, first rescuer gives one full slow breath
5. Second rescuer gives five chest compressions in 3–4 seconds (80–100/min), pauses for ventilations
6. First rescuer gives one slow full breath after each five compressions; checks compression effectiveness
7. Continue cycle (5 : 1) per step 13 above

Mouth to nose; mouth to stoma; bag valve mask; demand valve; EOA or airway inserted

Variations

Watch for gastric distension. Do not relieve it unless respirations are ineffective. Watch for vomiting and prepare to suction.

Caution

Do not interrupt CPR for more than 15 seconds.

Start O_2 as soon as possible.

Remember

Use jaw thrusts if cervical spine injury is suspected.

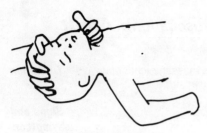

Open the airway

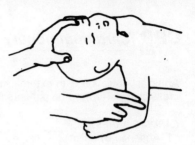

Check brachial pulse

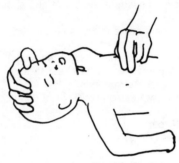

Chest compression, infant (1/2 to 1 in.)

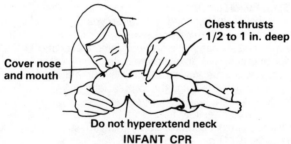

Cover nose and mouth

Chest thrusts 1/2 to 1 in. deep

Do not hyperextend neck

INFANT CPR

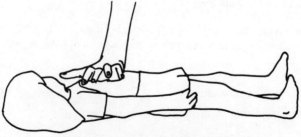

Chest compression, child (1 to 1 1/2 in.)

Artificial ventilation with external cardiac massage (chest compressions) performed on infants and children in cardiac arrest

Definition

1

Priority

CARDIAC ARREST
1. Absence of breathing
2. Absence of pulse

Signs and Symptoms

Follow same sequence as for adult CPR (p. 71) with these variations:
1. Airway
   a. Infant
      (1) Do *not* overextend the neck; a neutral position is best
2. Breaths
   a. Infant
      (1) Cover nose and mouth with your mouth
      (2) Give two slow full breaths, enough to make the chest rise
      (3) Give one full slow breath after every five compressions
   b. Child
      (1) Give one full slow breath after every five compressions
3. Pulse
   a. Infant
      (1) Use brachial pulse
4. Compressions
   a. Infant
      (1) Use two fingers only, one finger width below imaginary line between nipples
      (2) Depress ½–1 in
      (3) Rate, minimum 100/minute (5 per 3 seconds or less)
   b. Child
      (1) Use heel of one hand one finger width above sternal notch
      (2) Depress 1–1½ in
      (3) Rate, 80–100/minute (5 per 3–4 seconds)

Observe for gastric distension; do not attempt to relieve unless respirations are ineffective; prepare to suction.

Caution

Do not use demand valve resuscitators on children under 12 years of age unless the airway is severely compromised. Request medical direction. (Follow local protocol.)

Infant: newborn to 12 months; child: 1–8 years

Note

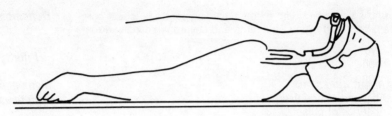

Oropharyngeal airway

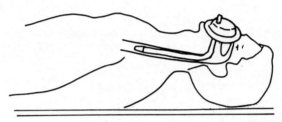

Esophageal obturator airway (EOA)

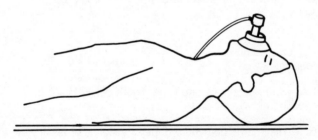

Demand valve

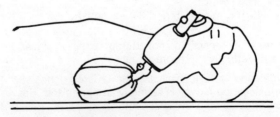

**Bag valve mask
(with O$_2$ reservoir)**

Mechanical Aids to Breathing

Devices placed into or over the airway to facilitate ventilation or the administration of oxygen to a patient   ***Definition***

ADJUNCT AIRWAYS   ***Types***
1. Oropharyngeal (inserted into mouth)
2. Nasopharyngeal (inserted into nostril)
3. Esophageal obturator airway (EOA) (inserted deep into the esophagus): follow local protocol

General rules for adjunct airways
1. Use only on unconscious, nonbreathing patients
   a. Nasopharyngeal airway can be used on a conscious patient
2. Measure for correct oropharyngeal airway size
3. Do not force tongue into throat on insertion
4. Remove when gagging, spitting, coughing, and breathing reflexes return
5. Use water soluble lubricant (K-Y Jelly) for nasopharyngeal and EOA airways
6. Prepare for vomiting and suction on removing airway

POSITIVE PRESSURE DEVICES
1. Demand valve
   a. Powered by tank pressure
   b. Automatic (patient demand) or manual (operator activated)
   c. Can be attached to some masks and adjunct airways
   d. Can deliver 100% O_2 at 100 lpm
   e. Do not use on children under 12 years of age. (Follow local protocol.)
2. Bag valve mask (Ambu bag)
   a. Manually powered (operator squeezes bag)
   b. Can be attached to O_2 supply
   c. Can deliver 100% O_2 with reservoir attached
   d. Can be attached to EOA or endotracheal tube

Follow local protocol for the use of EOA.   ***Note***

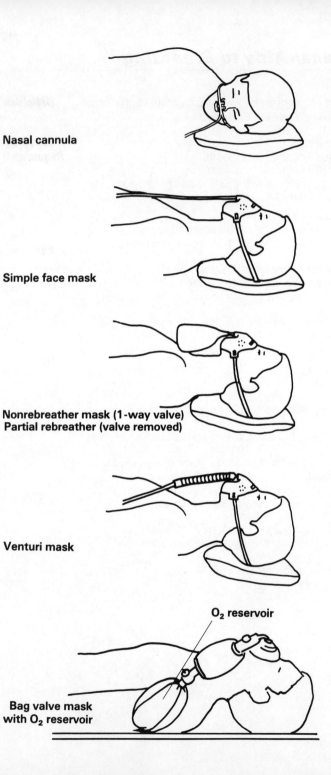

Nasal cannula

Simple face mask

Nonrebreather mask (1-way valve)
Partial rebreather (valve removed)

Venturi mask

O_2 reservoir

Bag valve mask
with O_2 reservoir

Oxygen Therapy

The administration of supplemental oxygen (O_2) to patients requiring supportive respiration

Definition

Airway obstruction	Respiratory distress	
Artificial ventilation	Seizure	
Cardiac arrest (MI)	Shock	
Chest pain	Stroke (CVA)	
Chest trauma	Toxic fumes, smoke, carbon	
Drowning	monoxide inhalation	
Respirations below 10/min	Unconsciousness	

Conditions Requiring O_2

Nasal cannula; face mask; partial rebreather mask; nonrebreather mask; venturi mask; bag valve mask; flowmeter; O_2
source

Equipment

Delivery device and flow rate (liters/minute) determine O_2 concentration; patient's condition determines device and rate.

Rates

Delivery Device	O_2 Concentration	Flow rate
Nasal cannula	24%–54%	1–6 lpm
Simple face mask	35%–60%	6–12 lpm
Partial rebreather	35%–60%	6–10 lpm
Nonrebreather	80%–95%	8–12 lpm
Venturi	24%–50%	4–12 lpm
Bag valve mask		
a. Without O_2	21% (normal air)	
b. With supplemental O_2	50%–100%	
Positive pressure (demand		
valve) resuscitator	100%	

Oxygen is a medication and is administered for a reason; know
the reason.

Warning

Watch patient for vomiting; be prepared to suction.

Monitor patient's breathing and O_2 flow.

O_2 dries mucous membranes. Humidify when administered 30
minutes or more. Follow local protocol.

Note

Explain to patient what you are doing and why.

Safety Precautions

Do not use oil or grease with O_2 equipment (cylinders, regulators, fittings, valves, hoses).

Do not smoke or use open flame when O_2 is in use.

Do not store or use O_2 in 125°F or higher environment.

Use only proper-fitting regulator valve assembly.

Close all valves when not in use.

Secure or protect tanks or cylinders from falling.

Never place yourself over valve assembly.

Always assure an adequate supply of O_2 on hand.

Inspect and maintain all O_2 equipment regularly.

Do not use equipment needing repair.

Use only oxygen labeled U.S.P. (United States Pharmacopeia)

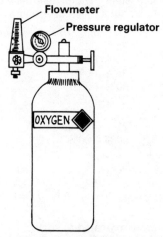

Flowmeter

Pressure regulator

OXYGEN

O_2 cylinder (green)

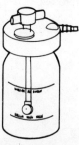

O_2 humidifier

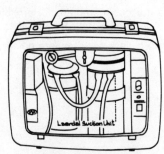

Portable suction unit

Oxygen Equipment

Components of oxygen delivery systems found on fixed, mo-
bile, and portable units

Definition

OXYGEN CYLINDER

Components

The oxygen cylinder (green in color) is a compressed (2000 psi)
source of O_2.

Size	Volume (liters)	Duration Constant	Duration/Max. Flow (15 lpm)
D	350	0.16	29 min
E	650	0.28	50 min
M	3000	1.56	4 h, 41 min

Calculate duration as follows:

$$\frac{(\text{gauge pressure} - 200) \times \text{constant}}{\text{flow rate (lpm)}} = \text{duration of flow (minutes)}$$

PRESSURE REGULATOR
The *pressure regulator* reduces tank pressure.
A *gauge* shows tank pressure remaining.
The *flowmeter* sets and shows flow rate (0 to 15 lpm).

HUMIDIFIER
The humidifier adds moisture to O_2, which is a drying agent.

SUCTION DEVICES
Suction devices are pumps for clearing the airway of blood,
vomitus, and secretions. They may be motor, manual, vacuum,
or compressed gas (O_2) powered, and may be fixed or portable.

Never respond without an adequate O_2 supply and working
delivery systems.

Warning

Do not suction longer than 15 seconds; watch for vomiting in
semiconscious and unconscious patients.

Caution

Close all valves when not in use.

Remember

Humidify O_2 when administered longer than 30 minutes. Follow
local protocol.

Traumatic Injuries

This section reviews traumatic injuries from head to toe, dressing, bandaging, and splinting.

Guidelines

1. Complete primary and secondary surveys are required to assess and treat an injuried patient properly.
2. **Signs and symptoms** listed here include most but not necessarily all the signs and symptoms of the named injury.
3. In general, the order of signs and symptoms is from high to low priority, most to least evident, and most to least common.
4. In general, signs and symptoms are grouped by relationship to a common organ, function, or other shared characteristic.
5. The presence of a sign or symptom, and *not* its place on the list, determines its significance in assessing an injury.
6. All, some, or no symptoms may be present.
7. **Treatment** described here refers to minimum suggested approved procedures by qualified personnel.
8. In general, the order of treatment is from the most to least urgent.
9. All injuries must be individually assessed and treated according to local standards and protocols.

This section will help you to

1. Identify, assess, and treat the named injuries.
2. Prepare for transport and transport injuried patients.

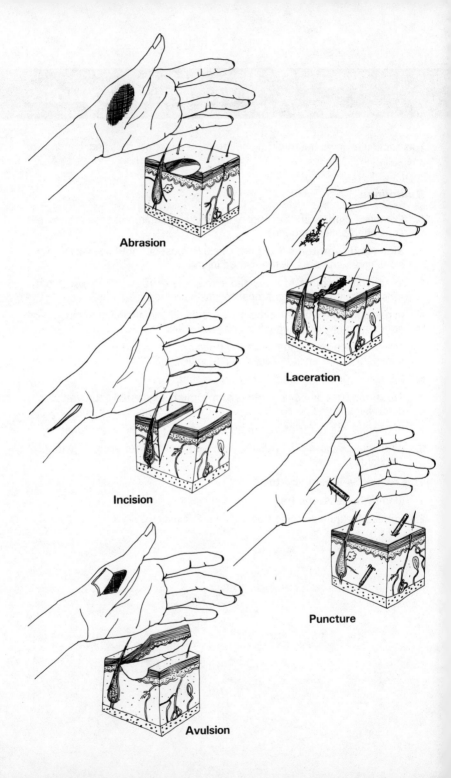

Abrasion

Laceration

Incision

Puncture

Avulsion

Soft Tissue Injury

1, 2, 3 (determined by severity of injury)   *Priority*

Physically caused damage to the skin and underlying muscles,   *Definition*
tendons, ligaments, cartilage, blood vessels, and nerves

OPEN   *Categories*
Skin is broken.   *and Classes*
1. Abrasion: skin is scraped away
2. Incision: sharp, even tissue cut
3. Laceration: torn, jagged wound (cut or tear)
4. Puncture: penetration by a narrow object
5. Avulsion: tissue separation by tearing

CLOSED
Skin is unbroken.
1. Contusion (bruise: skin discoloration due to subcutaneous bleeding
2. Internal laceration: internal cut or tear
3. Internal puncture: internal penetration
4. Crush injury: violent squeezing
5. Rupture: internal tear or break

1. Maintain airway; assist breathing (if required)   *Treatment*
2. Expose wound; clear surface foreign matter only
3. Control bleeding: use direct pressure, elevate, ice, pressure point, air splint, MAST, or tourniquet
4. Secure impaled objects: use bulky dressings
5. Apply dry, sterile dressing
6. Immobilize injured part
7. Elevate injured part, if possible
8. Check distal pulse
9. Calm patient
10. Transport

Transport patient in position of comfort unless nature and severity of injuries require a specific transport posture.   *Transport*

Prevent further wound contamination.   *Note*

Determine history of blood disorders, anticoagulant medication.

Large bruises may mean serious blood loss.

Always look for entrance and exit wounds of penetrating injuries.

Save avulsed parts.

Methods of Bleeding Control

1. Direct pressure over injury site
2. Elevation of affected extremity or part
3. Pressure points on major arteries
4. Ice or cold pack on injury site
5. Tourniquet above injury (last resort only, notify ER)

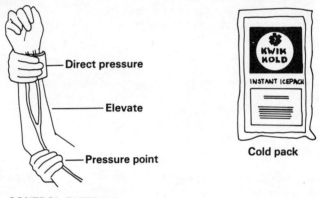

Direct pressure

Elevate

Pressure point

CONTROL BLEEDING

Cold pack

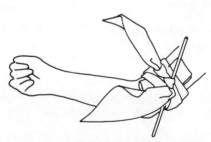

Tourniquet (last resort)

Bleeding

1, 2, 3 (determined by severity of injury)	**Priority**

The flow of blood from arteries, veins, or capillaries — **Definition**

Arterial: bright red, spurting, pulsing flow from an artery — **Types**
Venous: dark red, steady flow from a vein
Capillary: slow, even flow or oozing from capillaries

INTERNAL (Inside Body) — **Signs and Symptoms**
1. Bloody vomit, urine, sputum, stool
2. Rectal and vaginal bleeding
3. Signs and symptoms of shock
4. Abdominal tenderness, rigidity, spasms, guarding
5. Penetrating skull injuries
6. Blood in ears and nose
7. Large bruises, especially on abdomen
8. Fractured bones, especially long bones

EXTERNAL (Outside Body)
1. Visible bleeding

INTERNAL — **Treatment**
1. Treat for shock and administer O_2
2. Anticipate vomiting
3. Loosen tight clothing
4. Apply pressure dressing to injured extremity
5. Give nothing by mouth

EXTERNAL
1. Maintain airway
2. Control bleeding
3. Elevate legs
4. Splint fractures
5. Monitor patient and treat for shock

Transport in position of comfort or as injury/condition requires. — **Transport**

Determine history of hemophilia, blood disorders, or anticoagulant therapy. — **Note**

Head injury, chest injury, abdominal injury, pelvic fracture, and femur fracture produce internal bleeding. — **Remember**

Signs of Rising Intracranial Pressure

1. Deteriorating level of consciousness
2. Hemiplegia or quadriplegia
3. Vomiting
4. One pupil dilates (both if bilateral injury)
5. Rising blood pressure or decreasing pulse rate
6. Apnea or abnormal respirations

Cheyne-Stokes Breathing

Alternating periods of apnea and deep, rapid breaths

Head Injury Categories

Minimal: Alert and talkative; mild contusion possible
Moderate: Closed injury without head pain, little or no loss of consciousness or confusion
Severe: Coma, decerebrate, decorticate, flaccid

Points to Remember

1. Treat head injuries as spine injuries until disproven.
2. The most important sign of a head injury is a changing level of consciousness.
3. A head injury does not cause shock; look for another cause when shock is present.
4. Hypoxia is the most common cause of death in a head-injured patient; *do not* fail to secure and maintain the airway and administer O_2.
5. Monitor and record neurologic signs accurately and frequently.
6. *Do not* perform nasal suctioning if CSF fluid is present.
7. Alcohol and drugs may mask serious injuries

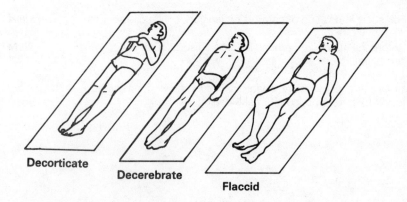

Decorticate

Decerebrate

Flaccid

Head Injury

Priority

Physical trauma to the scalp, skull, or brain   *Definition*

Types

Scalp	*Skull*	*Brain*
Laceration	Fracture	Concussion
Hematoma	Puncture	Contusion
Avulsion		Hematoma
Burn		Hemorrhage

Signs and Symptoms

BRAIN INJURY
1. Simple to severe headache
2. Disorientation, confusion, garbled speech
3. Breaks, deformities, depressions in skull
4. Rising blood pressure, falling pulse
5. Unequal pupils, eyes deviate, eye sunken
6. Vomiting, incontinence
7. Vision or hearing impairment
8. Blood or clear fluid from nose or ears
9. Asymmetrical facial movement
10. Limb paralysis, rigidity, decorticate or decerebrate positioning
11. Change from irritable to irrational behavior
12. Changing level of consciousness; unconsciousness
13. Bruising or swelling under eyes or behind ears
14. Breathing pattern changes (Cheyne-Stokes)

Treatment

1. Maintain airway; assist breathing; give O_2
2. Control bleeding cautiously
   a. Do *not* plug ears or nose
   b. *No* pressure bandages over head fractures
3. Immobilize cervical spine
4. Monitor vital signs and level of consciousness
5. Treat for shock; do not overheat
6. Keep patient awake; give emotional support

Transport

Conscious, no neck or spine injury: Semi-Fowler's
Unconscious or coma, no neck or spine injury: Coma
Unconscious or coma, with neck or spine injury: Supine on
   longboard; watch for vomiting; tip and suction

Warning

Sudden loss of consciousness or change in the level of consciousness is a true emergency.

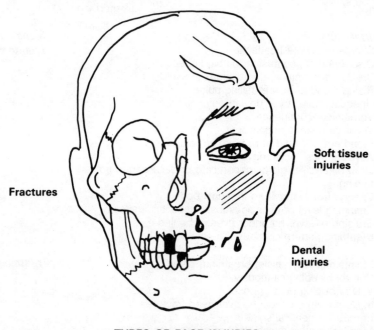

Fractures

Soft tissue injuries

Dental injuries

TYPES OF FACE INJURIES

Face Injuries

1 (major trauma); 3 (minor trauma)   *Priority*

Trauma to facial bones and tissue   *Definition*

FRACTURES   *Types*
1. Orbital (eye socket, cheek)
2. Nasal (broken nose)
3. Maxillary (upper jaw)
4. Mandibular (lower jar)

SOFT TISSUE
1. Bleeding
2. Lacerations, contusions, hematomas
3. Puncture (impaled objects)
4. Avulsions (nose, ears, lips, tongue, cheeks)
5. Burns (see p. 210, 217)

DENTAL
1. Broken or avulsed teeth

1. Visible bleeding, wounds, bruises, burns   *Signs and*
2. Visible swelling, deformities, nose deflected   *Symptoms*
3. Eye fixed and unable to move

1. Secure airway; examine for broken teeth and dentures   *Treatment*
2. Assist breathing and administer O_2
3. Remove impaled object from cheek
4. Control bleeding and dress open wounds
5. Immobilize head, neck, or lower jaw when indicated
6. Watch for vomiting; prepare to suction
7. Treat for shock

Semi-Fowler's (when there is no spine injury)   *Transport*
Coma position (when airway is compromised)

Assume cervical spine injury with massive facial trauma.   *Remember*

Do *not* hyperextend neck if spinal injury is suspected.

Save avulsed teeth and tissue for reimplantation.

Blunt forehead injury may cause behavior changes.   *Note*

Airway obstruction, shock, brain, and spine injury.   *Look for*

Special Considerations

Assume a serious head injury if signs and symptoms of fractured eye orbit are present.
1. Swelling at site; sunken eyeball
2. Double vision; pain on looking up
3. Reduced sensation of affected side cheek
4. Blood in nostril of affected side or under conjunctiva (mucous membranes of eye)
5. Eye deviated downward and inward
6. Unable to elevate or move eye

General Rules for Eye Care

1. *Never* apply any pressure to eye (including rubbing, touching, massaging, scratching by patient)
2. Do not apply medications to eye
3. Do not remove blood or blood clots from eye
4. Do not force eyelid except for irrigation
5. Continue irrigation throughout transport
6. Use only tepid water or saline solution to irrigate
7. Avoid unnecessary use of injured eye
8. Wash your hands before treating eye injuries
9. Always explain to patient what you are doing

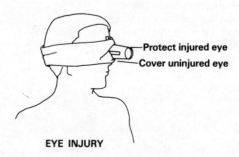

Protect injured eye
Cover uninjured eye

EYE INJURY

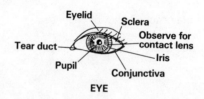

Eyelid
Sclera
Observe for contact lens
Tear duct
Iris
Pupil
Conjunctiva

EYE

Eye Injuries

1, 2, 3 (determined by severity of injury)	*Priority*

Physical trauma to the eyeball, orbit, conjunctivae, and lids *Definition*

1. Foreign object *Types*
2. Laceration, abrasion, contusion, avulsion, puncture, bleeding
3. Burns (heat, chemical, light)

1. Visible foreign object *Signs and*
2. Visible laceration, abrasion, contusion, avulsion, puncture *Symptoms*
3. Visible burn
4. Swollen or distorted eyeball
5. Bloodshot sclera (white portion of eyeball)
6. Pain or tenderness
7. Abnormal gaze, blurred or double vision
8. Orbital bruise ("black eye")
9. Orbital instability

1. Examine for physical injury and foreign bodies *Assessment*
2. Examine for eye motion
  a. Do eyes move together?
  b. Do they move in all directions?
  c. Is there pain on movement?
3. Examine pupils
  a. PERLA (*P*upils *E*qual, *R*eactive to *L*ight, *A*ccommodating)
  b. Blood overlying iris
4. Examine for visual acuity (ask patient to report)
  a. Blurred or double vision
  b. Light flashes, blocked visual field, dark spots

1. Flush immediately if chemical burns *Treatment*
2. Remove contact lenses (follow local protocol)
3. Flush away chemicals and foreign objects with water or saline solution for minimum of 20 minutes
4. Cover damaged eye with moist dressing
5. Cover avulsed or impaled eye with protective cup
6. Tape uninjured eye closed (unconscious patient only)
7. Patch both eyes to limit movement if eyeball is damaged

Semi-Fowler's (supine if retina is detached), low light; transport *Transport*
avulsed eyelid pieces (sterile dressing, ice)

Do *not* apply pressure or force when treating eye. *Remember*

Frequent Causes of Spinal Injury

1. Motor vehicle accidents
2. Falls
3. Diving accidents
4. Cave-in, structure collapse
5. Lifting heavy objects
6. Related severe head or face injury
7. Any major trauma
8. Lightning injury

Complications of Spinal Injury

1. Injury to C1–C4 compromises or stops breathing
2. Injury to C4–C7 produces diaphragmatic breathing
3. Neurogenic shock, death
4. Paralysis

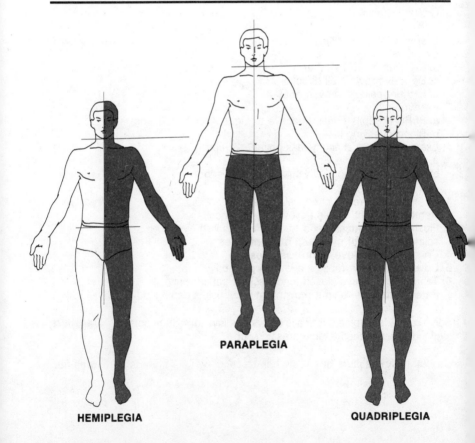

PARAPLEGIA

HEMIPLEGIA

QUADRIPLEGIA

Spinal Injuries

1 (with respiratory distress); 2	**Priority**

Physical trauma to the spinal cord or column — **Definition**

Fracture (vertebrae) **Types**
Rupture (disk)
Squeeze, crush, stretch, tear, or severing (spinal cord)

Signs and Symptoms

1. Spinal pain, tenderness, deformity with or without movement
2. Numbness, weakness, heaviness in extremities
3. Impaired or diaphragmatic breathing
4. Asymmetrical or absent reflexes
5. Hypotension
6. Bradycardia
7. Incontinence
8. Priapism (obvious in children, less in adults)
9. Muscle spasms along spine
10. Unconscious with flaccid muscles
11. Paralysis (most reliable sign)
    a. Hemiplegia (one side [usually head injury, CVA])
    b. Paraplegia (lower extremities)
    c. Quadriplegia (all extremities)

Assessment

1. Consider mechanism of injury
2. Observe patient position
3. Perform thorough secondary survey and sensory tests
4. Monitor patient for changes

Treatment

1. Immobilize patient (*do not move* unless airway is impaired; remove helmet if airway is compromised. Follow local protocol.)
   a. Head: extrication or rigid collar
   b. Spine: long board, scoop, short board
2. Assist breathing, give high concentration O_2
3. Monitor for changes, observe for vomiting
4. Suction

Supine (longboard), proceed slowly and gently — **Transport**

Warning

Respiratory failure from spinal injury can cause death.

Assist ventilations if needed.

Do *not* hyperextend neck; use chin or jaw lift if patient needs CPR.

Always assume spinal injury if mechanism of injury suggests it. — **Remember**

Frequent Causes of Neck and Throat Injuries

1. Motor vehicle accidents
2. Crushing blow
3. Fall
4. Strangulation (accidental or deliberate)
5. Hanging (suicide attempt or accidental)

Note

1. Do *not* apply pressure to both sides of neck at the same time or over airway.
2. Do *not* place bandage around neck; use tape to hold dressings in place.
3. Make certain an occlusive dressing over severed vein injury is airtight to guard against air embolism.

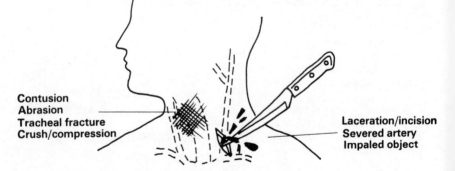

Contusion
Abrasion
Tracheal fracture
Crush/compression

Laceration/incision
Severed artery
Impaled object

TYPES OF SOFT TISSUE INJURIES

Neck and Throat Injuries (*Soft Tissue*)

1, 2, 3 (determined by severity of injury)	**Priority**

Open or closed trauma to trachea, larynx, blood vessels, nerves, skin, muscles, and tissue of the neck **Definition**

1. Laceration, incision   5. Severed vein   **Types**
2. Abrasion   6. Crush, compression
3. Contusion   7. Impaled object
4. Tracheal fracture

1. Visible bleeding, bruise, tissue damage, swelling, depres- **Signs and**
   sion, deformity (especially Adam's apple) **Symptoms**
2. Obstructed airway, impaired breathing
   a. Shortness of breath
   b. Changes or loss of voice
   c. Respiratory stridor (high-pitched sound)
   d. Drooling (cannot swallow)
3. Subcutaneous emphysema (crackling when palpated)
4. Frothy, bloody foam from wound or mouth
5. Pain and tenderness

TRACHEAL FRACTURE **Treatment**
1. Immobilize cervical spine; avoid handling
2. Administer O_2 (high concentration)
3. Reassure patient and instruct him to breath slowly
4. Apply cold pack

TRACHEA OR LARYNX LACERATION
1. Secure airway
2. Control bleeding
3. Administer O_2 (high concentration)
4. Suction airway

SEVERED VEIN
1. Place patient in left lateral recumbent position, head down
   10 to 15 degrees
2. Control bleeding above and below injury site
3. Place occlusive dressing over wound
4. Support breathing (O_2, 10 to 12 lpm, nonrebreather)

Semi-Fowler's position if tracheal injury; coma position (left **Transport**
lateral recumbent) if severed neck vein

Always look for cervical spine injury. **Note**

Lung Sounds

1. Rales indicate fluid in bronchioles and alveoli
     Fine: crackling sound
     Medium: medium-pitched bubbling or gurgling
     Coarse: lower pitched bubbling or gurgling
2. Rhonchi indicate thick secretions, muscular spasm, external pressure
     Sound: continuous, rumbling, more harsh than rales
3. Wheezes indicate narrowed airways
     Sound: high-pitched whistling

Complications

**Signs and
Symptoms**
CARDIAC TAMPONADE
1. Distended neck veins
2. Falling blood pressure, increasing shock
3. Distant or hard-to-hear heart sounds

Treatment
1. ABC's, stabilize patient
2. Administer O_2, treat shock, MAST (follow protocol)
3. Transport: Fowler's; *do not delay*

**Signs and
Symptoms**
RUPTURED AORTA
1. Sudden, severe chest pain
2. Signs and symptoms of shock
3. Absent or delayed femoral pulse

Treatment
1. ABC's, stabilize patient, administer O_2
2. *Transport at once (true emergency)*

**Signs and
Symptoms**
TRAUMATIC EMPHYSEMA
1. Chest pain, respiratory distress, cyanosis
2. Weakness, paralysis, convulsions, unconsciousness
3. Coughing, impaired vision

Treatment
1. ABC's, stabilize patient
2. Administer O_2
3. Transport: semi-Fowler's position

Common Causes of Chest Injury

1. Motor vehicle accidents
2. Blunt trauma
3. Cave-in, structure collapse

Chest Injuries (*General*)

1, 2, 3 (determined by severity of injury)	**Priority**
Open or closed trauma to skin, tissue, bone, blood vessels, nerves, and organs of the thorax	**Definition**

Types

1. Laceration, incision   **4.** Crush, compression
2. Abrasion, contusion   **5.** Puncture, sucking
3. Bone (rib) fracture   **6.** Impaled object

Signs and Symptoms

1. Visible trauma, bleeding, bruises
2. Pain or tenderness on palpation
3. Respiratory distress, painful breathing, coughing
4. Weak, rapid pulse
5. Hypotension
6. Cyanosis
7. Coughing bright red, frothy blood (punctured lung)
8. Distended neck veins or deviated trachea
9. Chest fails to expand and contract normally
10. Paradoxical chest movement
11. Unequal air entry on auscultation with stethoscope

Assessment

1. Look for visible injury, breathing symmetry
2. Listen for equal right and left lung sounds, sucking air, clear heartbeat
3. Feel for breathing symmetry, rib and rib cage instability, crackling air under skin

Treatment

1. Secure and maintain airway
2. Assist breathing; 100% O_2 (use demand valve if required)
3. Control bleeding
4. Monitor, control for shock, apply MAST (follow protocol)
5. Cover sucking chest wounds with occlusive dressing
6. Splint ribs
7. Stabilize impaled object in place
8. Stabilize flail chest segment
9. Monitor breathing pattern changes and vital signs
10. Prepare to suction vomit, blood, secretions

Transport

Semi-Fowler's position; place patient on injured side if breathing is easier

Caution

Be alert for complications (see opposite page).

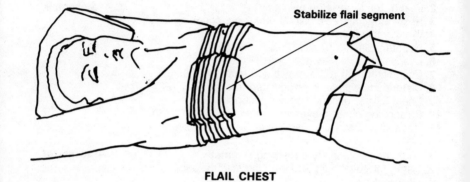

Stabilize flail segment

FLAIL CHEST

Flail Chest

1   *Priority*

The separation of a free segment of chest wall caused when   *Definition*
several consecutive ribs fracture in two places, or separation of
the sternum from the ribs, allowing paradoxical (opposite) chest
motion

1. Respiratory distress (shallow, rapid)   *Signs and*
2. Pain on breathing or reluctance to breath deeply   *Symptoms*
3. Paradoxical movement of flail (free) segment
4. Cyanosis possible
5. Tachycardia possible
6. Decreased breath sounds

1. Secure and maintain airway   *Treatment*
2. Support respiration; administer 100% O_2
   a. Mask if breathing is adequate
   b. Demand valve if breathing inadequate
   c. Encourage deep breathing
3. Stabilize flail segment
4. Treat for shock
5. Monitor vital signs
6. Watch for signs of heart or lung injury

Semi-Fowler's position if no shock; lay patient on affected side   *Transport*
if more comfortable. Transport rapidly.

Flail chest may be accompanied by lung and heart injuries (lac-   *Warning*
erations, punctures, contusions).

Breathing problems and hypoxia can cause rapid deterioration
and are an immediate threat to life.

Use demand valve *only* if risk of no O_2 exceeds possible pres-   *Caution*
sure-induced pneumothorax.

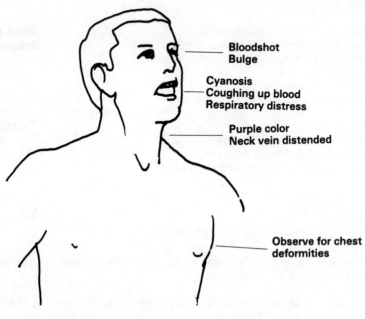

Bloodshot
Bulge

Cyanosis
Coughing up blood
Respiratory distress

Purple color
Neck vein distended

Observe for chest
deformities

TRAUMATIC ASPHYXIA

Traumatic Asphyxia

1; a **true emergency**

Sudden, severe compression to the chest or the upper abdomen, forcing blood from the right side of heart (wrong way) into neck, head, and shoulder veins; it may also cause severe lung damage (ruptured alveoli)

1. Deep blue or purple color in head, neck, shoulders
2. Cyanosis (nail beds, lips, tongue, skin)
3. Respiratory distress (shortness of breath)
4. Pain at injury site; increases with breathing
5. Eyes are bloodshot and protruding (bulging)
6. Coughing up blood; bloody vomitus
7. Chest fails to expand normally on inspiration
8. Chest deformities
9. Hypotension
10. Severe shock
11. Pulse rapid and weak
12. Upper body edema
13. Face, neck, and shoulder veins are distended

1. Secure and maintain airway
2. Assist breathing; demand valve, administer 100% O_2
3. Control external bleeding
4. Treat for shock; apply MAST (follow local protocol)
5. Monitor airway; prepare to suction
6. Monitor vital signs, respirations

Immediate transport; position determined by severity of injury; notify ER

Primary goal is to keep patient alive; watch carefully for deterioration.

Traumatic asphyxia indicates massive injury; it may be associated with flail chest and rib fractures.

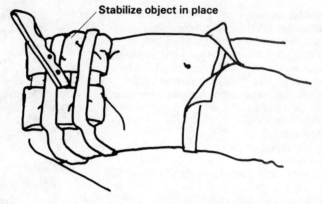

Stabilize object in place

IMPALED OBJECT

Object Impaled in Chest

1 — **Priority**

Penetration of the chest wall by any object that remains embedded — **Definition**

Signs and Symptoms
1. Visible impaled object
2. Respiratory distress, painful breathing, coughing
3. Pain or tenderness on palpation
4. Weak, rapid pulse
5. Hypotension
6. Cyanosis
7. Unequal right and left lung sounds, sucking air
8. Coughing bright red frothy blood

Treatment
1. Do *not* remove object
2. Stabilize object in place
3. Assist breathing, administer O_2 (high concentration)
4. Control bleeding with direct pressure
   a. Do *not* touch object
   b. Do *not* apply pressure near cutting edge
5. Treat for shock, apply MAST (follow local protocol)

Position that best guards object from touch and movement — **Transport**

Use extreme care to limit movement to avoid increasing hemorrhage, pain, and shock when it is essential to shorten a long impaled object. — **Warning**

Sanitary napkins make excellent bulky dressings. — **Note**

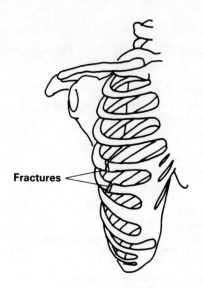

Uncomplicated rib fracture

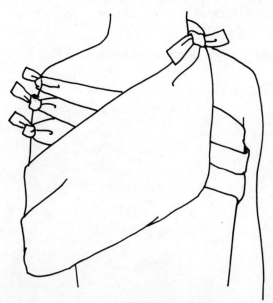

Rib fracture splint

Fractured Ribs

1 (complicated); 2 (uncomplicated)	*Priority*

A partial or complete break in one or more ribs   *Definition*

Uncomplicated: little or no bone displacement   *Classification*
Complicated: visible depression, open wound, external bleeding; sucking sounds; internal bleeding

UNCOMPLICATED   ***Signs and***
1. Pain on breathing, coughing, moving, touch at site   ***Symptoms***
2. Patient leans forward, splints ribs with hand or arm
3. Shallow breathing

COMPLICATED
1. Above signs and symptoms, with
2. Visible depression, open wound, bleeding
3. Internal bleeding, coughing bloody froth
4. Sucking sounds, unequal lung sounds
5. Crackling under skin on palpation

UNCOMPLICATED   ***Treatment***
1. Immobilize fracture site; not too tightly
2. Assist breathing; administer O_2 (40%; nasal cannula)

COMPLICATED
1. Bandage bleeding wounds, apply occlusive dressing if
   sucking wound; use pillow to support and splint site
2. Treat for specific injury
   a. Flail chest (p. 99)
   b. Traumatic asphyxia (p. 101)
   c. Pneumothorax (p. 107)

Semi-Fowler's; lay patient on affected side.   *Transport*

Presume damage or danger to underlying organs, and treat   *Caution*
accordingly.

Loosen binding if breathing is difficult when bound.   *Note*

Patient often can pinpoint injury site.

Treatment

SIMPLE PNEUMOTHORAX
1. Secure and maintain airway
2. Administer O_2 and assist breathing as required
3. Sit patient in Fowler's position unless related injuries prohibit
4. Transport at once

SUCKING CHEST WOUND
1. Secure and maintain airway
2. Administer 100% O_2 (10–12 lpm; nonrebreather)
3. Seal open chest wound with occlusive dressing (apply at end of forced exhalation)
4. Monitor for changes in breathing and vital signs; unseal dressing if there is deterioration; reseal as required during transport
5. Transport at once on affected side

TENSION PNEUMOTHORAX
1. Secure and maintain airway
2. Administer 100% O_2; assist ventilations
3. Unseal dressing if tension pneumothorax is result of sucking wound
4. Transport at once on affected side

HEMOTHORAX
1. Secure and maintain airway
2. Administer O_2 (high concentration); assist ventilations as required
3. Control external bleeding
4. Treat for shock; apply MAST (follow local protocol)
5. Transport at once on affected side

Caution   If pulse pressure (difference between systolic and diastolic pressure) decreases steadily, assume a serious chest cavity injury. A pulse pressure below 15 mmHg is critical.

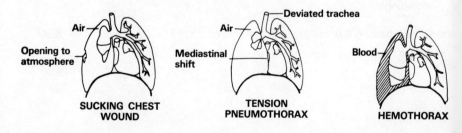

SUCKING CHEST WOUND   TENSION PNEUMOTHORAX   HEMOTHORAX

1; a **true emergency**   *Priority*

Lung collapse due to air or blood entering the pleural space   *Definition*

SIMPLE PNEUMOTHORAX: air enters pleural space from hole   *Types*
in lung

SUCKING CHEST WOUND: air enters pleural space from hole in
chest wall to atmosphere.

TENSION PNEUMOTHORAX: air trapped in pleural space com-
presses heart and opposite lung.

HEMOTHORAX: blood enters pleural space.

SIMPLE PNEUMOTHORAX   *Signs and*
1. Respiratory distress   *Symptoms*
2. Trachea deviation toward injured side
3. Sudden, sharp pain in chest
4. Chest movement on affected side stops
5. Tachycardia, weak pulse, hypotension
6. Diaphoresis, pallor, elevated temperature
7. Dizziness, anxiety
8. Hollow percussive chest sound on affected side
9. Diminished breathing sounds on affected side

SUCKING CHEST WOUND
1. Signs and symptoms for simple pneumothorax with
2. Visible and audible chest wound
3. Frothy, bright red blood in mouth

TENSION PNEUMOTHORAX
1. Signs and symptoms for simple pneumothorax with
2. Extreme respiratory distress, high voice
3. Deviated trachea, distended neck veins
4. Subcutaneous emphysema (crackling under skin)
5. Breathing sounds absent on affected side

HEMOTHORAX
1. Signs and symptoms for simple pneumothorax with
2. Signs of hemorrhagic shock

See opposite page.   *Treatment*

Pneumothorax: Fowler's; hemothorax, pneumothorax: lay pa-   *Transport*
tient on affected side

Treatment
Principles
1. Prevent soft tissue damage from swelling
   a. Remove or cut rings, jewelry, clothing distal to injury
2. Control bleeding; dress or bandage wounds
3. Support or hold traction until immobilized and splinted
4. Do *not* straighten spine, shoulder, elbow, wrist, knee, ankle fracture; *splint as found*
5. Do *not* retract or push bone ends under skin
6. Immobilize joints above and below fracture site
7. Check distal pulses *before* and *after* splinting and bandaging
8. Splint firmly but do *not* impair circulation
9. Do *not* move patient before all fractures or dislocations are immobilized
10. Do *not* apply traction in crush injuries or if ankle is fractured/dislocated (follow local protocol)

Treatment
SPRAIN/STRAIN
1. Treat related injuries and conditions
2. Immobilize and splint
3. Apply ice pack
4. Transport as required, in position of comfort

DISLOCATION
1. Treat related injuries and conditions
2. Evaluate distal pulse, temperature, capillary refill, neurovascular status
3. Immobilize and splint in position found
4. Reevaluate distal limb status, per step 2
5. Apply ice pack
6. Transport in position of comfort

FRACTURE
1. Treat related injuries and conditions
2. Evaluate distal pulse, temperature, capillary refill, neurovascular status
3. Apply traction as required (follow protocol); immobilize and splint
4. Reevaluate distal limb status, per step 2
5. Apply ice pack
6. Transport in position of comfort

Forces Producing Skeletal Injury

1. Direct force (injury occurs at contact site)
2. Indirect force (injury occurs away from contact site)
3. Twisting force
4. Violent muscular contractions
5. Repeated stress
6. Pathological effects/effects of aging

Musculoskeletal Injuries (*General*)

2, 3   *Priority*

Physical trauma to bones, cartilage, ligaments, muscles or tendons   *Definition*

Fracture: bone break   *Types*
Dislocation: joint separation
Sprain: tendon, muscle, ligament overstretch or tear
Strain: muscle tear, overstretch

Ask for   *Assessment*
1. Mechanism of injury, direction of force
2. Location of pain, tingling, numbness
3. Movement of part (*no* if neck or spine injury)

Look for
1. Deformity, swelling, discoloration
2. Shortening; unnatural or absent motion (paralysis)
3. Visible bone ends or open wound

Evaluate for
1. Point tenderness and nerve impairment
2. Distal pulses and capillary fill

SPRAIN/STRAIN	*DISLOCATION*	*Signs and*
1. Pain, tenderness	1. Pain (worse if moved)	*Symptoms*
2. Swelling, redness	2. Tenderness, swelling	
	3. Deformity	
	4. Loss of motion	

FRACTURE
1. Patient heard break
2. Point tenderness, pain, guarding
3. Swelling, bruising
4. Deformity, unnatural motion, loss of use
5. Extremity shortened
6. Crepitus (grating sound), exposed bone ends

See opposite page.   *Treatment*

Position of comfort   *Transport*

Treat the whole patient when treating a fracture: airway, breathing, bleeding, dress wounds, treat shock.   *Remember*

Blood vessel, nerve, and soft tissue damage in a fracture is more significant than the fracture.

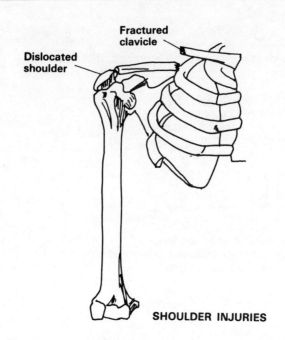

Fractured clavicle

Dislocated shoulder

SHOULDER INJURIES

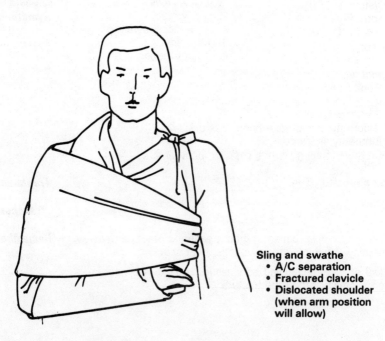

Sling and swathe
- A/C separation
- Fractured clavicle
- Dislocated shoulder
  (when arm position
  will allow)

Shoulder Injuries

3   *Priority*

Dislocated shoulder, acromion/clavicle (A/C) separation, or frac-   *Definition*
tured clavicle

1. "Dropped" shoulder (injured side shoulder is lower than   *Signs and*
   uninjured; droops forward)   *Symptoms*
2. Patient splints injured arm across chest; holds injured side
   elbow with uninjured side hand
3. Inability or refusal to raise arm
4. Clavicular pain
5. Point tenderness
6. Clavicular deformity, swelling, lumps
7. Bruising
8. Crepitus (grating sound; if fracture)
9. Distal numbness

1. Seat or have patient lie down   *Treatment*
2. Support arm
3. Apply cold pack
4. Sling and swathe; position of comfort; pad or pillow under
   upper arm; don't let forearm droop
5. Check distal pulse before and after splinting
6. Watch for fainting
7. Nothing by mouth

Position of comfort; semi-Fowler's   *Transport*

Do *not* minimize clavicle injury; rib fracture and subsequent   *Caution*
lung and blood vessel injury is common.

Never attempt to reduce shoulder dislocation.

If dislocation reduces itself, treat as above and transport; patient must be examined by physician.

Transport as soon as possible if absence of distal pulses.

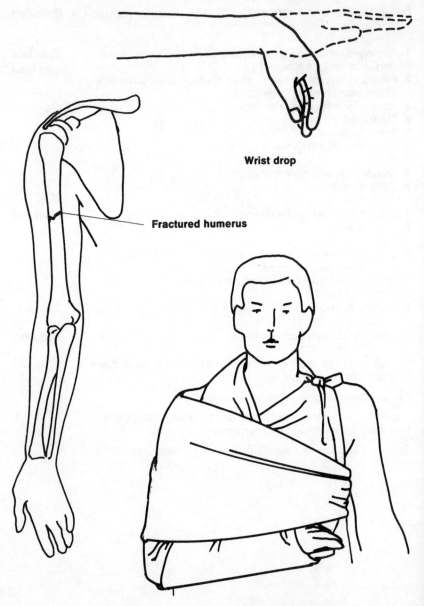

Wrist drop

Fractured humerus

Sling and swathe

Humerus

1 (open fracture), 3 (closed fracture)	*Priority*

A fracture of the humerus — *Definition*

Signs and Symptoms
1. Point tenderness
2. Deformity or angulation
3. Swelling, bruising at site
4. Loss, hesitation of use
5. Crepitus (grating sound)
6. Exposed bone (open fracture)
7. "Wrist drop"
8. Numbness or tingling

Treatment
1. Control bleeding (open fracture)
2. Dress or bandage wound
3. Check distal pulse; if none, extend elbow slightly and re-check
4. Splint and immobilize; padded board or ladder splint; sling and swathe
5. Recheck distal pulse and capillary fill; if none, transport immediately
6. Apply cold pack to site
7. Observe for swelling, discoloration, cold extremity

Transport
Semi-Fowler's; recheck distal pulse, capillary fill, swelling, discoloration

Caution
If flexing arm stops circulation, immobilize with elbow straight or reposition gently to obtain pulse.

"Wrist drop" indicates radial nerve involvement

Remember
When splinting, leave fingertips and radial pulse accessible.

Note
Remove rings, watches, bracelets to other extremity.

Distal humerus fracture is often accompanied by nerve and blood vessel damage, and is serious.

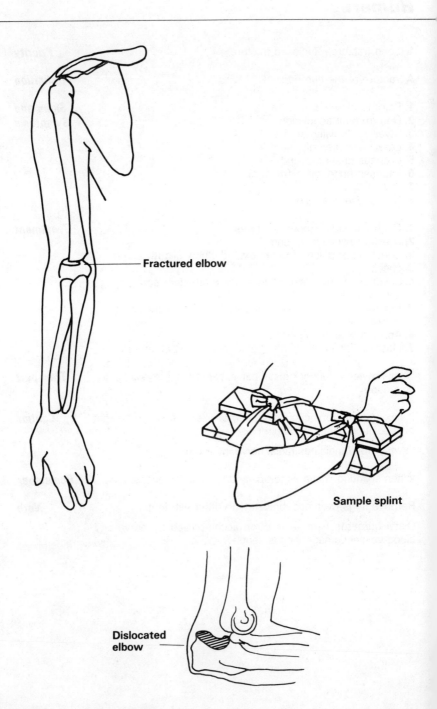

Fractured elbow

Sample splint

Dislocated elbow

2   *Priority*

Fracture or dislocation of the elbow joint, the hinged articulation   *Definition*
of the humerus, radius, and ulna

1. Pain, swelling, point tenderness   *Signs and*
2. Pain is made worse on movement   *Symptoms*
3. Deformity
4. Loss of motion; patient refuses to move
5. Decreased circulation to hand

IF ARM IS BENT   *Treatment*
1. Do *not* straighten
2. Assess distal pulse and nerves; if no pulse, *gently* try to
   reposition *one time only*
3. Sling and swathe
4. Assess distal pulse, nerves, temperature
5. Cold pack

IF ARM IS STRAIGHT
1. Do *not* bend
2. Assess distal pulse, nerves, temperature
3. Place pad under armpit
4. Splint elbow with well-padded splint or pillow splint
5. Assess distal pulse, nerves
6. Cold pack
7. Lay patient down; elevate injured arm

Semi-Fowler's/supine, with arm elevated on pillows.   *Transport*

Do *not* force elbow into anatomical position.   *Caution*

If from a fall on extended arm, look for wrist fracture and radial   *Note*
head fracture

When uncertain, treat an elbow injury as a fracture.

Wire ladder splints and padded board splints are effective for   *Remember*
elbow injuries.

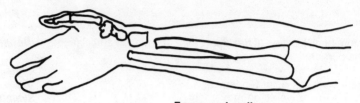

Fractured radius

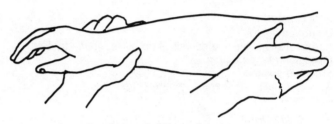

Gentle traction if angulated

Position of function

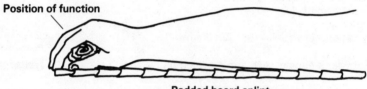

Padded board splint
Immobilize above and below fracture

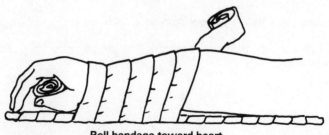

Roll bandage toward heart

TREATMENT PROCEDURE

Forearm (*Radius/Ulna*)

2 (open); 3 (closed)	**Priority**

Fracture of the radius or ulna — **Definition**

Signs and Symptoms
1. Deformity, angulation
2. Crepitus (grating sound)
3. Pain, point tenderness
4. Bleeding, swelling, bruising
5. Inability or unwillingness to move arm
6. Exposed bone ends (open fracture)

Treatment
1. Control bleeding (open fracture)
2. Dress or bandage wound
3. Severe angulation
   a. Straighten carefully with gentle traction
   No or minimal angulation
   a. Splint as found
4. Splint with well-padded splint; splint with hand in position of function; immobilize joints above and below fracture
5. Assess distal pulse and nerve
6. Sling and swathe
7. Cold pack

Transport
Position of comfort (semi-Fowler's); elevate arm if patient is supine

Note
Remove rings, watches, jewelry to opposite arm.

Severe deformity or angulation indicates likelihood of radius *and* ulna fracture.

Remember
Monitor for distal neurovascular status, capillary refill, and swelling before and after splinting.

A closed, one-bone forearm fracture may produce pain and tenderness, but little or no deformity.

Forearm fracture usually results from a fall on outstretched hand.

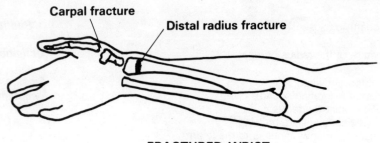

FRACTURED WRIST

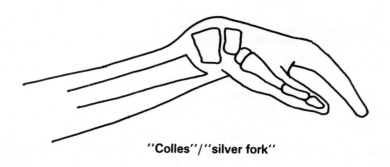

"Colles"/"silver fork"

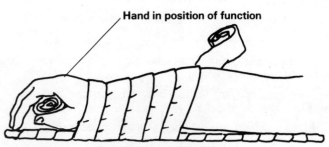

Roll bandage toward heart

TREATMENT PROCEDURE

Wrist

3   *Priority*

Dislocation or fracture at the articulation of the radius, ulna, and   *Definition*
hand

1. Pain, point tenderness   *Signs and*
2. Swelling, deformity   *Symptoms*
3. "Colles" or "silver fork" appearance
4. Inability or unwillingness to move extremity

1. Assess distal pulse and nerve function   *Treatment*
2. If deformed, straighten gently
3. Splint in position of function; hand roll; padded board
    splint; pillow; sling and swathe
4. Assess distal pulse and nerve function
5. Apply ice pack

Position of comfort or supine with injured extremity elevated by   *Transport*
sling and swathe or pillow.

Air splints reduce swelling.   *Note*

Remove rings, watches, and jewelry to opposite extremity.

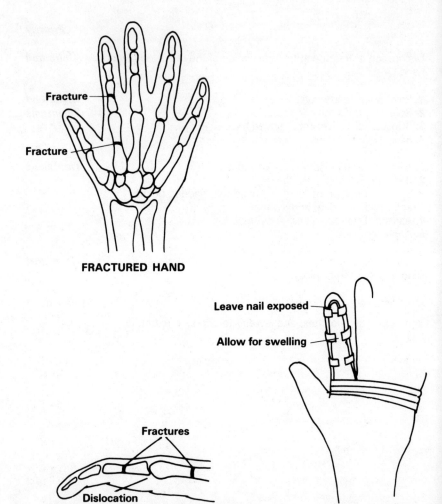

FRACTURED HAND

FINGER FRACTURES AND DISLOCATION

FINGER SPLINT

Hand/Finger

1 (crush injury); 3 (uncomplicated injury)	*Priority*

Fracture or dislocation of the bones of the hand   *Definition*

1. Visible bleeding, open wounds, exposed bone, swelling   *Signs and*
   deformity   *Symptoms*
2. Acute pain, point tenderness
3. Limited or no finger movement

CRUSH INJURY   *Treatment*
1. Do *not* cleanse wounds
2. Put ball of soft cloth in patient's palm
3. Splint and bandage entire hand in position of function
4. Bandage fingers separately if possible, use nonadhering
   bandage
5. Support with sling and elevate to prevent swelling
6. Observe for impaired circulation and swelling
7. Leave fingertips exposed to assess circulation

CLOSED FRACTURE (*Single Finger*)
1. Splint with padded splint in position of function
2. Elevate and sling

Position of comfort   *Transport*

Watch for massive swelling; splint, dress, bandage, and sling   *Caution*
accordingly; keep hand elevated at heart level.

Do *not* reduce dislocated fingers.

Splint hand/finger injuries in position of function.   *Note*

Splints: tongue depressor; adjoining fingers; aluminum finger
splint; board splint; foam rubber

Transport amputated parts to ER.   *Remember*

Remove rings, watches, and jewelry to opposite extremity/
hand.

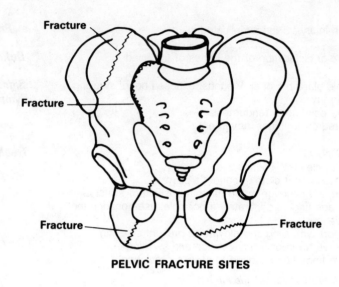

PELVIC FRACTURE SITES

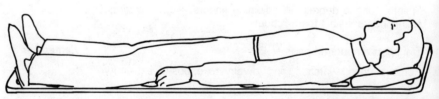

**Immobilize with longboard
Apply straps as required**

Pelvis

1	*Priority*

Fracture of the bones of the pelvic girdle	*Definition*

1. Compress hip bones medially | *Assessment*
2. Press pubic bones
3. Have patient squeeze your fist between his knees

1. Pain, especially with above assessment | *Signs and*
2. Point tenderness | *Symptoms*
3. Bruising
4. Deformity
5. Unwillingness to move legs
6. Spasm of lumbar spine muscles
7. Crepitus (grating sound)
8. Abdominal pain
9. Blood in urine or around urethra opening
10. Shock

1. *Minimize movement* | *Treatment*
2. Place on back; *log roll*
3. Bind folded blanket between legs with wide cravats;
   splint with MAST (follow local protocol)
4. Assess femoral pulses for equality
5. Immobilize on longboard or scoop stretcher
6. Administer O_2
7. Flex knees and support with pillow (to reduce pain)
8. Monitor vital sings, neurovascular status; watch for shock

Supine; *handle gently; rapid* transport | *Transport*

Puncture of bladder and internal organs of pelvic cavity, hemor-rhagic shock, lumbosacral spine injury, and associated lower extremity fractures make this injury a serious threat to life. | *Caution*

Blood loss from pelvic fracture may be extensive. | *Warning*

Shock commonly occurs with multiple pelvic fractures.

Pelvic fracture is difficult to detect; note mechanism of injury. | *Note*

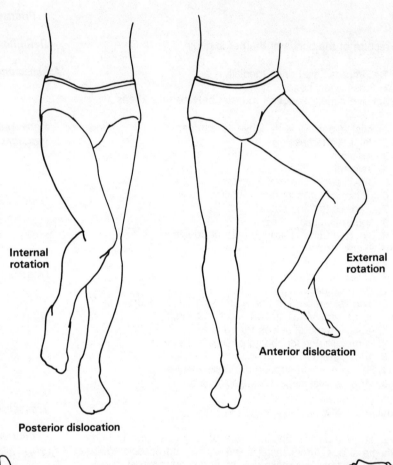

Internal rotation

External rotation

Anterior dislocation

Posterior dislocation

Immobilize with longboard
Apply straps as required

Hip

Priority

The fracture or dislocation of the head of the femur **Definition**

FRACTURE **Signs and**
1. Pain at site and proximal groin; sometimes at knee **Symptoms**
2. Pain and tenderness on pressing greater trochanter (prominence at head of femur)
3. Bruising, swelling, discoloration at site
4. Supine patient can't lift affected limb
5. Injured side foot turned out
6. Affected limb appears shortened

DISLOCATION
1. Intense pain
   a. Anterior dislocation (less common)
      (1) Entire affected limb rotated outward.
   b. Posterior dislocation (more common)
      (1) Knee bent, limb rotated inward, appears shortened
      (2) Foot hangs loose ("foot drop")
      (3) Patient can't flex foot or lift toes
      (4) Loss of sensation in affected limb

1. Assess neurovascular function **Treatment**
2. Bind folded blanket between legs with wide cravats in position found, or
3. Apply traction splint (follow local protocol), or
4. Apply MAST (follow protocol)
5. Place on long board or scoop stretcher
6. Monitor for shock; administer O_2 as required
7. Monitor neurovascular function
8. Apply cold pack; cushion with pillows

Position of comfort; support and cushion affected limb; *handle* **Transport**
gently

Do *not* reduce dislocation; notify ER of spontaneous reduction. **Caution**

Heavy internal bleeding is possible; monitor shock.

Even minor trauma or a simple fall may produce hip fracture in **Remember**
elderly.

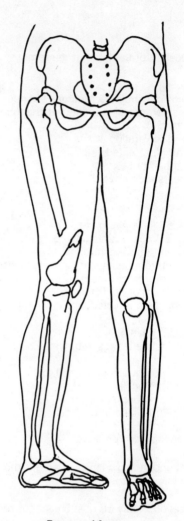

Fractured femur

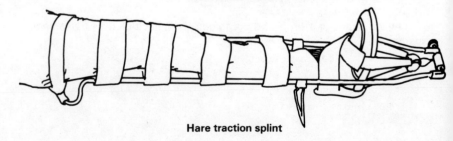

Hare traction splint

Femur

1 *Priority*

A closed or open fracture of the femur *Definition*

1. Severe pain, point tenderness, crepitus (grating sound) *Signs and*
2. Swelling, deformity, exposed bone ends *Symptoms*
3. Loss of pulse, feeling, function below fracture
4. Foot turned out
5. Muscle spasms, injured leg shortened
6. Shock

1. Control bleeding; dress and bandage wound *Treatment*
2. Immobilize injured leg
   a. Splint
      (1) Traction unless fracture 1 to 1½ in from knee (follow local protocol)
      (2) MAST, long leg, blanket
3. Check distal pulse and nerve function before and after splinting
4. Monitor vital signs
5. Treat for shock; administer O_2 as required
6. Ice pack

Position of comfort *Transport*

Loss of distal pulse requires immediate transport. *Caution*

Do *not* overlook related life-threatening injuries.

Do *not* apply traction if
Crush injury
Ankle/tibula–fibula dislocation
Fracture within 1½ in of the knee

A femur injury may suggest spinal or other injury. *Note*

Assume 1–2 l blood loss in a closed fracture.

Follow local protocol regarding the use of traction splinting. *Remember*

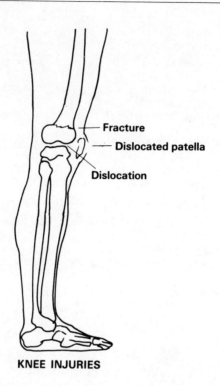

KNEE INJURIES

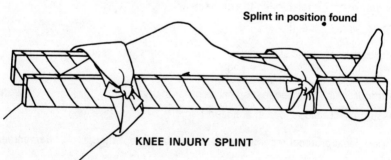

Splint in position found

KNEE INJURY SPLINT

Knee

2   *Priority*

Fracture, strain, sprain, or dislocation of the bones or connec-   *Definition*
tive tissue of the knee joint

1. Pain, tenderness   *Signs and*
2. Deformity, angulation, patella displaced   *Symptoms*
3. Rapid swelling
4. Inability to move joint
5. Crepitus (grating sound)

1. Assess neurovascular function   *Treatment*
   a. If pulse, do *not* straighten
   b. If *no* pulse, try to straighten *one time only;* do *not* force
2. Immobilize in position found with rigid, pillow, blanket, air,
   or padded splint
3. Assess neurovascular status
   a. If signs of impairment, transport at once
4. Apply cold pack

Position of comfort; pad and support affected leg.   *Transport*

Popliteal artery damage or impairment poses a serious threat to   *Caution*
the injured limb; monitor closely.

Treat and transport spontaneously reduced patella dislocation
as if unreduced; notify ER.

Fractures, dislocations, and torn cartilage are difficult to distin-   *Note*
guish; treat the same.

The knee is a highly complex joint; treat with care.   *Remember*

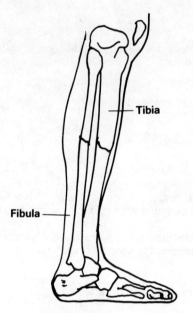

TIBIA AND FIBULA FRACTURES

Include knee and ankle joints in splint

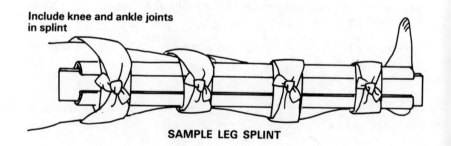

SAMPLE LEG SPLINT

Tibia/Fibula

1 (open); 2 (closed)   *Priority*

Fracture of the tibia or fibula   *Definition*

CLOSED   *Signs and*
1. Pain, point tenderness   *Symptoms*
2. Swelling
3. Deformity, angulation
4. Crepitus (grating sound)
5. Unwillingness to move leg

OPEN
1. All of the above, with
2. Open wound, bleeding
3. Visible bone ends

1. Control bleeding (open fracture)   *Treatment*
2. Dress and bandage wounds or apply cold packs
3. Assess distal pulse and nerve function
4. Gently correct severe angulation with steady manual traction
5. Apply splints to both sides of leg; padded board, air, three-
sided cardboard box, traction, or bind to other leg with
blanket between legs
6. Assess distal pulse and nerve function

Position of comfort; elevate leg if possible   *Transport*

If *no* distal pulse and nerve function, transport at once; no- *Caution*
tify ER.

Do *not* let bone ends penetrate skin.

Include knee and ankle joints in splint.   *Note*

Follow local protocols when using traction splint.

Impairment of nerve and blood supply is a serious emergency. *Remember*

Severe deformity or angulation is common.

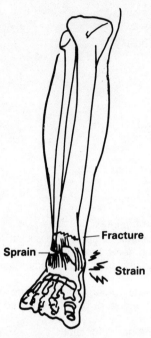

ANKLE INJURIES

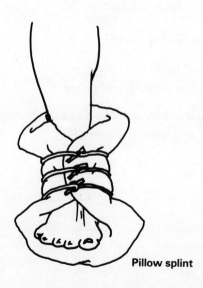

Pillow splint

Ankle

2   *Priority*

Fracture, sprain, strain, or dislocation of the bones and tissues   *Definition*
of the ankle joint

1. Pain, point tenderness, pain on rotation   *Signs and*
2. Rapid swelling   *Symptoms*
3. Deformity
4. Unwillingness to move foot or bear weight

1. Lay patient down and remove his shoes   *Treatment*
2. Assess distal pulse and nerve function
    a. If none, gently straighten deformity with steady longitu-
       dinal traction
3. Elevate limb
4. Dress open wounds
5. Splint with pillow, air, padded board, figure 8 bandage
6. Assess distal pulse and nerve function
7. Apply cold pack

Semi-Fowler's or supine; support injured leg with pillows   *Transport*

Do *not* straighten angulation if distal pulse is present.   *Caution*

Do *not* let injured foot dangle; elevate.

Treat all ankle injures as fractures.   *Note*

If using a padded rigid splint, splint from above knee to below
foot; mold and bandage pillow splint around foot and ankle.

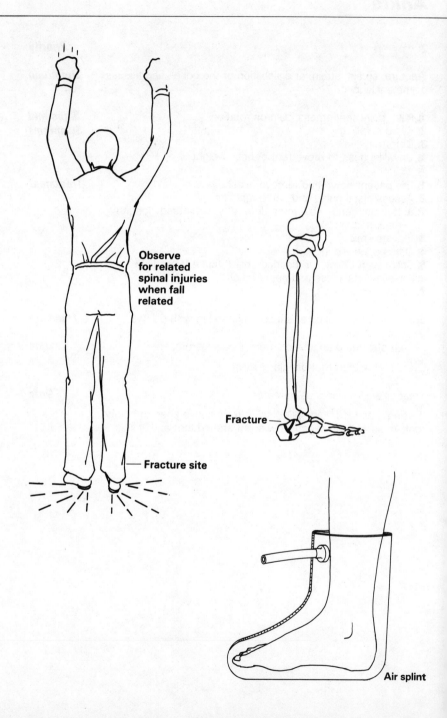

Observe for related spinal injuries when fall related

Fracture site

Fracture

Air splint

3   *Priority*

Fracture, sprain, strain, dislocation, or soft tissue injury to bones, connecting tissue, and soft tissue of the foot and toes   *Definition*

1. Visible bleeding, wounds, punctures   *Signs and Symptoms*
2. Pain
3. Deformity (toe injury; uncommon with foot injury)
4. Swelling (severe in crush injury)
5. Inability to bear weight
6. Tiptoe limp (heel injury)
7. Bruising under heel (heel, foot, toe injury)
8. Crepitus (grating sound)

1. Control bleeding   *Treatment*
2. Dress and bandage wounds
3. Assess pulse and nerve function
4. Elevate injured extremity
5. Splint; pillow or air splint; splint broken toe with tape to adjoining toe
6. Monitor pulse and nerve function
7. Apply cold pack

Position of comfort; injured leg elevated and supported, knee straight; do *not* let foot dangle.   *Transport*

A fall onto heels from a height of 15 feet or more is often associated with lumbar spinal injuries; splint spine with longboard.   *Caution*

Allow for swelling when splinting.   *Note*
Always check distal pulse and nerve function before and after splinting.

Associated Injuries

Chest wounds
Fractured ribs; punctured lung
Pelvis, middle or lower back injuries

Common Causes

Motor vehicle accident
Fall from height
Blunt trauma
Bullet, knife, penetrating injuries

Complications

Ruptured bladder, bowel, diaphragm
Hemorrhage; shock
Internal organ damage or bruising
Fractured pelvis, ribs, spine

Note   Do *not* remove impaled object or replace evisceration.

Pain may be referred; look for primary injury site.

Observe contents of vomitus.

Hemorrhage and shock are the major threats to life.

Look for exit wounds in penetrating or gunshot injuries.

Apply moist dressing and cover with occlusive dressing if abdominal evisceration (follow local protocol).

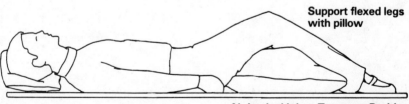

Support flexed legs with pillow

Abdominal Injury Transport Position

Abdominal Trauma (*General*)

1	*Priority*

Traumatic open or closed injury to the tissues and organs of the abdomen and abdominal cavity — *Definition*

Assessment

Look for	*Feel for*	*Listen for*
Bleeding	Tenderness	Bowel sounds
Wounds	Rigidity	
Bruises	Throbbing mass	
Distension		

Signs and Symptoms

1. Visible bleeding, wounds, bruises, distension
2. Pain at site or referred; mild, becoming severe
3. Cramps, nausea
4. Weakness
5. Thirst
6. Rapid, shallow breathing
7. Rapid pulse
8. Low blood pressure (starting high if severe pain)
9. Rigid or tender abdomen
10. Coughing up blood
11. Patient very still; legs drawn up; guards abdomen
12. Absent bowel sounds
13. Shock, anxiety
14. Vomiting
15. Blood in urine, from rectum or urethra

Treatment

1. Lay patient on back with legs flexed
2. Secure and maintain airway
3. Administer O_2; assist ventilations if required
4. Control external bleeding; dress and bandage wounds
5. Treat for shock; apply MAST (follow protocol)
6. Monitor vital signs
7. Be alert for vomiting; give nothing by mouth

Supine; legs flexed; *rapid* — *Transport*

Symptoms may be masked by other injuries; observe mechanism of injury. — *Caution*

Do *not* remove penetrating objects or touch eviscerated organs.

See facing page. — *Note*

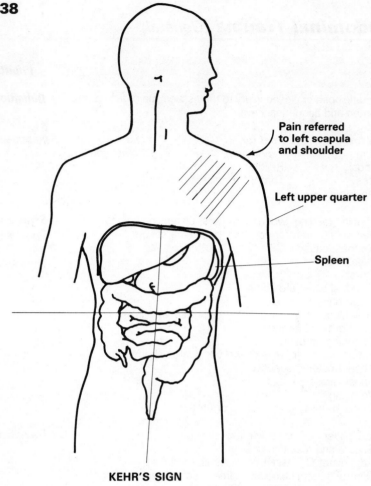

Pain referred to left scapula and shoulder

Left upper quarter

Spleen

KEHR'S SIGN

Common Causes

Blunt trauma
Motor vehicle accident
Falls
Bullet, knife, and penetrating injuries

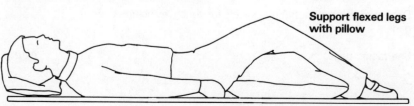

Support flexed legs with pillow

Abdominal Injury Transport Position

Ruptured Spleen

1 **Priority**

Traumatic injury to the spleen **Definition**

1. Abdominal pain; upper left quarter, radiating to left scapula **Signs and**
   and shoulder (Kehr's sign) **Symptoms**
2. Abdominal rigidity
3. Signs of internal bleeding
4. Rapidly developing shock
   a. Restlessness
   b. Pale, ashen color
   c. Rapid, shallow breathing
   d. Cyanosis
   e. Rising pulse
   f. Falling blood pressure
5. Patient guards abdomen

1. Lay patient on back with legs flexed **Treatment**
2. Secure and maintain airway
3. Administer O_2; assist ventilations as required
4. Monitor vital signs
5. Apply MAST as required (follow local protocol)
6. Nothing by mouth

Supine/most comfortable, with legs flexed; *rapid* **Transport**

Shock develops rapidly when spleen is ruptured. **Warning**

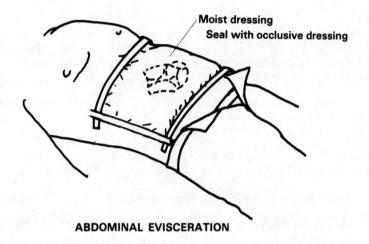

ABDOMINAL EVISCERATION

Abdominal Evisceration

1 *Priority*

Traumatic injury to the abdominal wall, exposing internal organs **Definition**

1. Visible open wound with exposed internal organs *Signs and*
2. Pain *Symptoms*
3. Bleeding
4. Rapid, shallow breathing
5. Rapid pulse
6. Patient guards abdomen
7. Increasing thirst
8. Shock

1. Lay patient on back with legs flexed *Treatment*
2. Assure and maintain airway; administer O_2, high concentration (nonrebreather)
3. Cut away clothing to expose wound
4. Do *not* touch protruding organs; do *not* attempt to replace them into abdominal cavity
5. Cover exposed organs with sterile dressing *soaked in sterile saline solution,* then cover dressing with multitrauma or universal dressing and seal with aluminum foil or plastic wrap (Saran) to conserve heat (follow local protocol)
6. If moist dressing unavailable, cover wound with nonadherent dressing such as aluminum foil, Saran Wrap, or other occlusive material (follow local protocol)
7. Treat for shock; apply MAST (check local protocol)
8. Monitor vital signs
9. Give nothing by mouth

Supine with legs flexed; *rapid* *Transport*

Do *not* handle exposed organs. *Caution*

Do *not* replace them into abdominal cavity.

Cover them with moist sterile dressing *only.*

Conserve body heat.

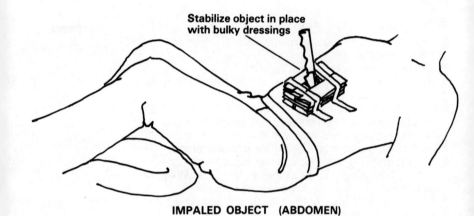

Stabilize object in place with bulky dressings

IMPALED OBJECT (ABDOMEN)

1   *Priority*

Penetrating wound to the abdomen with or without invasive   *Definition*
object left in place

1. Visible impaled object or puncture wound   *Signs and*
2. Visible bleeding   *Symptoms*
3. Pain
4. Patient guards abdomen
5. Shock
6. Internal bleeding
7. Ecchymosis (bruising) in flanks (sides between ribs and hips)
8. Absence of either or both femoral pulses

1. Lay patient on back with legs flexed   *Treatment*
2. Assure and maintain airway
3. Control bleeding
4. Administer O_2 (high concentration)
5. If impaled object
   a. Do *not* remove
   b. Stabilize in place
6. If penetrating wound
   a. Look for exit wound
7. Treat for shock; apply MAST, leg sections only (follow local protocol)
8. Monitor vital signs
9. Anticipate vomiting
10. Give nothing by mouth

Supine, legs flexed; *rapid*   *Transport*

Do not move or apply any pressure to impaled object; stabilize   *Caution*
securely in place.

If object must be shortened to facilitate transport, stabilize securely while cutting.

Death may be imminent; prepare to perform CPR.

Observe for exit wounds and other nearby wounds.   *Note*

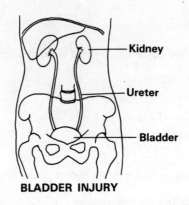

BLADDER INJURY

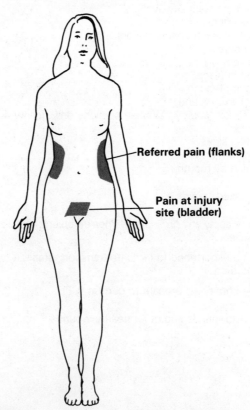

Referred pain (flanks)

Pain at injury site (bladder)

RADIATING PAIN OF RUPTURED BLADDER

Bladder (*Rupture/Laceration*)

1 | *Priority*

Rupture or laceration of the bladder usually is associated with pelvic fracture or blunt trauma to abdomen. Also, ruptured urethra is common with straddle injury. | *Definition*

BLADDER INJURY | *Signs and*
1. Signs and symptoms of abdominal/pelvic injury | *Symptoms*
2. Pain above pubis; may radiate to flank
3. Blood in urine (hematuria)
4. Difficult urination
5. Bladder spasms
6. Shock

URETHRA INJURY (*Straddle Injury*)
1. Pain
2. Inability to urinate or intermittent stream when urinating

1. Treat for abdominal or pelvic injury if indicated | *Treatment*
2. Monitor vital signs
3. Treat for shock
4. Keep patient at rest; reassure
5. Give nothing by mouth

Supine with legs flexed or position of comfort | *Transport*

Patient may not display symptoms for some time; they frequently are delayed. | *Note*

Also look for related urinary system problems if there is blood in urine.

Rapid deceleration of car with seat belt fastened may produce ruptured bladder. | *Remember*

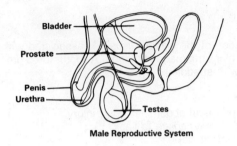

Male Reproductive System

Bladder

Prostate

Penis

Urethra

Testes

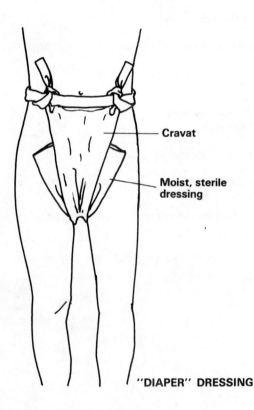

Cravat

Moist, sterile dressing

"DIAPER" DRESSING

Genital Injury (*Male*)

2	***Priority***

Traumatic injury to the penis, testicles, and scrotum	***Definition***

1. Visible bleeding or wound	***Signs and***
2. Intense pain	***Symptoms***
3. Swelling and bruising	

LACERATION, TEAR, OR AVULSION   ***Treatment***
1. Control bleeding
   a. Direct pressure
   b. Tourniquet to stump if amputation
2. Dress with moist, sterile dressing secured with cravat
   (diaper method)
3. Transport avulsed part in moist, sterile dressing

"FRACTURE" OR BLUNT TRAUMA
1. Treat open wounds as above
2. Apply ice pack to injured area

TESTICULAR TORSION   ***Special Case***
Spontaneous or injury-induced muscular spasm of spermatic
cord; usually occurs in patients 18 years old or younger

1. Sudden pain on affected side	***Signs and***
2. Sudden swelling or retraction of affected testicle	***Symptoms***
3. Tenderness of affected testicle	
4. Redness of scrotum	
5. Abdominal or back pain	

1. Apply ice pack to scrotum	***Treatment***
2. Transport as soon as possible (surgery imperative)	

Position of comfort	***Transport***

If genitalia are burned, keep area moist, transport patient at once.	***Caution***

Do not remove penetrating objects; stabilize.

Genital injuries are not necessarily life-threatening, but patient requires reassurance and privacy.	***Note***

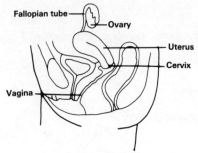

Female Reproductive System

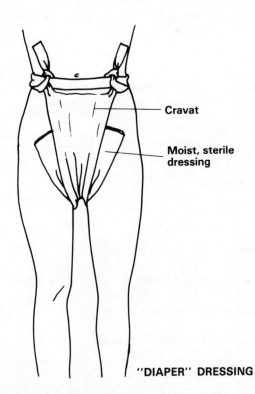

Cravat

Moist, sterile dressing

"DIAPER" DRESSING

Genital Injury (*Female*)

1 (ruptured uterus); 2 (other injuries) | ***Priority***

Traumatic injury to external soft tissues or internal reproductive organs | ***Definition***

1. Internal or external bleeding | ***Signs and***
2. Visible abrasion, laceration, avulsion | ***Symptoms***
3. Intense pain
4. Shock

1. Lay patient on back with legs flexed | ***Treatment***
2. Control bleeding
   a. Do *not* remove impaled objects
   b. Local pressure with moist, sterile dressing
   c. Do *not* place dressing in vagina
   d. Bandage dressing with cravat (diaper method)
3. Dress avulsed area with moist, sterile dressing
4. Apply cold pack (blunt trauma injury)
5. Administer O_2
6. Treat for shock
7. Apply MAST for ruptured uterus (follow local protocol)
8. Give nothing by mouth

RUPTURED UTERUS | ***Warning***
A true emergency

Indicated by profuse vaginal bleeding

Treat as above and transport *immediately*.

Supine; straddle injury, semi-Fowler's; ruptured uterus, rapid transport | ***Transport***

Never place dressings in vagina. | ***Caution***

Transport avulsed parts (rolled in moist sterile dressing, with fat side in).

All pregnant patients with injuries should be seen by a physician.

Administer O_2 to pregnant patients with injuries. | ***Note***

Maintain confidentiality and privacy. Be nonjudgmental in cases of rape. Allow patient to verbalize her feelings.

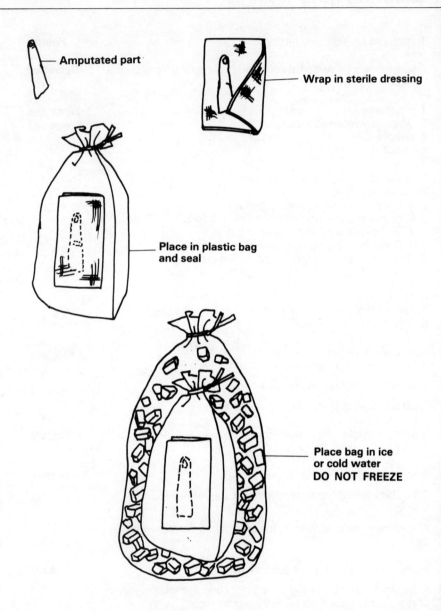

Amputated part

Wrap in sterile dressing

Place in plastic bag and seal

Place bag in ice or cold water
DO NOT FREEZE

Amputation

1, 2 (determined by severity)	*Priority*
Traumatic removal of body parts, limbs, or parts of limbs	*Definition*
1. Visible complete or partial removal of a body part	*Signs and Symptoms*

Treatment

1. Secure and maintain airway
2. Control bleeding
    a. Direct pressure
    b. Pressure points
    c. Tourniquet, as a last resort *only*
3. Elevate extremity
4. Dress stump with moist, sterile dressing
5. Monitor vital signs
6. Treat for shock; administer O_2 as required
7. Monitor closely for renewed bleeding
8. Locate and save amputated parts
    a. Wrap in sterile dressing
    b. Soak dressing with sterile saline
    c. Place in plastic bag and seal
    d. Place bag on ice or cold water; keep cool; do *not* allow tissue to freeze; label bag
    e. Transport with patient to ER
8. Remove rings, watches, jewelry from injured part

Transport

Position of comfort or as determined by extent and nature of injuries

Caution

Apply tourniquet *only* when all other methods to control bleeding have failed.

Do *not* loosen tourniquet once it has been applied.

Do *not* apply tourniquet to severed part.

Do *not* complete partial amputation.

Place severed part on sterile, gauze, saline-soaked dressing *only*; *no* antiseptic, *no* soap. (Follow local protocol.)

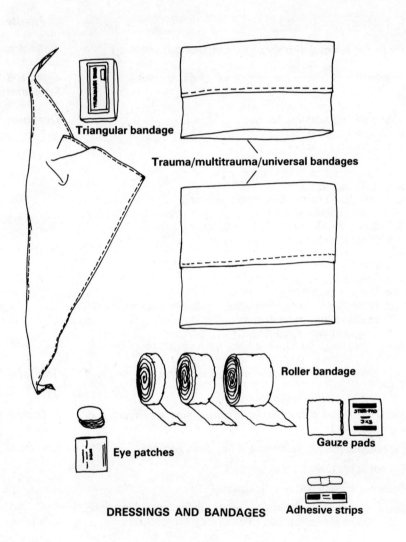

Triangular bandage

Trauma/multitrauma/universal bandages

Roller bandage

Eye patches

Gauze pads

DRESSINGS AND BANDAGES

Adhesive strips

Dressing/Bandaging

Dressings are any material (preferably sterile) used to cover a wound; bandages are any material used to hold dressings in place, but not to cover wounds. **Definition**

1. Control bleeding   **3.** Protect wounds   **Purpose**
2. Prevent contamination   **4.** Stabilize/immobilize

Aseptic: sterile (bacteria-free)   **Types**
Antiseptic: sterile (contain bactericide)
Wet: not always sterile
Dry sterile: sterile, moisture-free
Petroleum: sterile, soaked with petroleum jelly
Occlusive: airtight when sealed at edges
Adhesive: sterile, self-sticking

Adhesive strips/patches: small cuts, wounds   **Styles/Uses**
Roller bandage (rolled gauze): for securing large or small
    dressings, binding splints, immobilizing parts and objects
Trauma/universal/multitrauma dressings: for large injuries,
    bleeding control, stabilizing
Triangular bandage: sling, swathe, for securing large areas
    (head, chest, back, hip, buttocks, shoulder), binding splints,
    immobilizing

1. Expose wound or injured area   **Principles**
2. Handle sterile dressings by edges only
3. Cover entire wound plus surrounding area
4. Once applied, do *not* remove; add additional dressings and
    bandages on top of original
5. Leave fingers, toes, pulses exposed if possible
6. Monitor circulation *before* and *after* applying; loosen but do
    not remove if circulation stops
7. Secure loose ends

Check distal pulses *before* and *after* bandaging.   **Caution**

Wrap bandages toward the heart.

Do *not* use elastic bandages to secure dressings.

Remove rings and bracelets to opposite extremity.

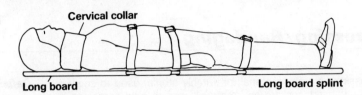

Cervical collar

Long board

Long board splint

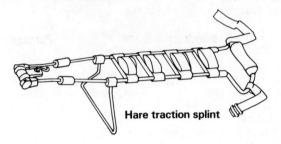

Hare traction splint

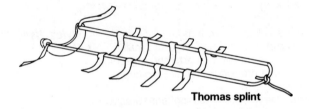

Thomas splint

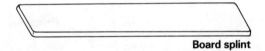

Board splint

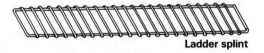

Ladder splint

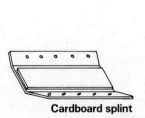

Cardboard splint

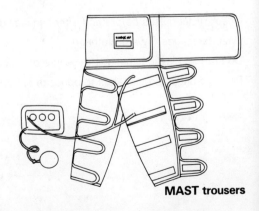

MAST trousers

Splinting

To immobilize, restrain, or support any body part with a rigid or flexible device   *Definition*

1. Immobilize broken bones and joints   *Purpose*
2. Prevent further tissue and nerve injury
3. Minimize pain and increase comfort
4. Prevent or reduce swelling and bleeding

Rigid: padded board, spine board, three-sided cardboard, ladder, cervical collar   *Types*
Soft: rolled blanket, pillow, cravats
Traction: commercial brands, half ring
Air: inflatable, vacuum

1. Locate and expose part to be immobilized   *Procedure*
2. Control bleeding; dress wounds
3. Straighten severely angulated fractures
4. Splint joints as found unless pulse absent
5. Assess distal pulse and nerve function *before* and *after* splinting
6. Secure splint above and below joint/fracture
7. Pad voids; cushion where possible
8. Leave distal pulses accessible
9. Apply cold pack
10. Elevate if possible

Immobilize fractures before moving the patient.   *Caution*

Do *not* push bone ends back into wound.

Inflate air splints *only* by mouth; not too stiff; acceptable if you can indent slightly with thumb.

Do *not* use traction splint on hip fracture in elderly patient. (Follow local protocol.)   *Note*

Work with a partner when splinting.

Inform patient what you are doing.

When in doubt, splint, and treat as a fracture.   *Remember*

This section reviews common medical emergencies in alphabetical order.

Guidelines

1. Complete surveys plus a medical history are required to properly assess and treat a patient needing medical care.
2. **Signs and Symptoms** listed here include most but not necessarily all the signs and symptoms of the named condition.
3. In general, the order of signs and symptoms is from high to low priority, most to least evident, and most to least common.
4. In general, signs and symptoms are grouped by relationship to a common organ, function, or other shared characteristic.
5. The presence of a sign or symptom and *not* its place on the list determines its significance in assessing a condition.
6. All, some, or no signs and symptoms may be present; they are intended only to aid patient assessment and may suggest a condition that requires evaluation by a physician.
7. **Treatment** described here refers only to minimum suggested approved procedures for use by qualified personnel.
8. In general, the order of treatment is from the most to least urgent.
9. All medical conditions must be individually assessed and treated according to local standards and protocols

This section will help you to

1. Identify, assess, and treat the named medical conditions.
2. Prepare for transport and transport medical patients.

Possible Conditions

Aortic aneurysm	Intoxication
Appendicitis	Kidney stone
Diabetic ketoacidosis	Mononucleosis
Diverticulitis	Ovarian cyst
Ectopic pregnancy	Pancreatitis
Fibroid uterine tumors	Ruptured uterus
Food poisoning	Sickle cell anemia
Incarcerated hernia	Ulcer
Intestinal obstruction	Ulcerative colitis
Gastroenteritis	Uremia

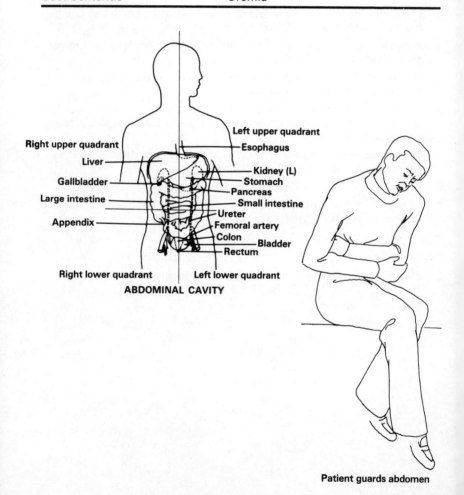

Left upper quadrant
Right upper quadrant
Esophagus
Liver
Kidney (L)
Gallbladder
Stomach
Pancreas
Large intestine
Small intestine
Ureter
Appendix
Femoral artery
Colon
Bladder
Rectum
Right lower quadrant
Left lower quadrant

ABDOMINAL CAVITY

Patient guards abdomen

Acute Abdomen

1   *Priority*

Acute onset of severe abdominal pain   *Definition*

1. Abdominal pain; local or diffuse   **Signs and**
2. Abdomen tender, soft, rigid, distended   **Symptoms**
3. Patient quiet, anxious, unwilling to move, guards abdomen
4. Tachycardia
5. Rapid, shallow breathing
6. Constipation, diarrhea, bloody (tarry) stools
7. Nausea, vomiting (bloody, "coffee-ground")
8. Diarrhea, constipation, bowel sounds
9. GI tract, penile or vaginal bleeding; bloody urine
10. Pulsating mass in abdomen (aortic aneurysm)
11. Hypotension
12. Shock
13. Fever

1. Secure and maintain airway   *Treatment*
2. Place patient on back with knees drawn up
3. Administer O_2 if respiratory distress
4. Monitor vital signs
5. Treat for shock
6. MAST (per orders; follow local protocol)
7. Nothing by mouth
8. Be prepared to suction

Position of comfort with knees drawn up; shock position   *Transport*

Acute abdomen may indicate a variety of conditions, many of   *Caution*
which are potentially life threatening; do *not* delay transport to
diagnose.

Abdominal conditions are difficult to assess. When in doubt,   *Note*
transport the patient to the hospital for evaluation.

Common Causes of Acute Asthma

Infections: Common cold, viral infections, sinusitis, bronchitis, bronchiolitis

Inhaled allergens: Pollens (weeds, grasses, trees), house dust, animal fur, feathers, molds, mildews

Inhaled irritants: Paints, solvents, gasoline, perfume, tobacco smoke, industrial chemicals, air pollution, cold air

Food allergies: Milk, eggs, chocolate, nuts, fish, shellfish, strawberries, tomatoes

Trigger mechanisms: Physical exertion, temperature changes, laughter, emotional reactions, nasal polyps

Drugs: Penicillin, vaccines, aspirin, anesthetics, other drugs

Psychological stress: Stress, anxiety, tension

Acute Asthma

1	<div align="right">***Priority***</div>

Marked episodic respiratory distress due to spasm, swelling, or secretions in the bronchus
Definition

1. Respiratory distress (mild to severe); audible with stethoscope
2. History of asthma
3. Patient sitting up, leaning forward
4. Anxiety, fighting for breath, wheezing
5. Cough (productive or unproductive)
6. Overinflated chest; use of accessory muscles to breathe; increased breathing rate
7. Pursed lips
8. Cyanosis (mild) of nailbeds and lips
9. Patient drowsy (DANGER)
10. Silent chest (DANGER)
11. Tachycardia
12. Slightly elevated blood pressure

Signs and Symptoms

1. Secure and maintain airway
2. Keep patient sitting up
3. Administer *humidified* O_2; be prepared to ventilate
4. Monitor vital signs
5. Maintain calm reassurance
6. Assist with prescribed medications

Treatment

Fowler's, semi-Fowler's, position of comfort; RAPID
Transport

Obtain immediate history to rule out other causes, especially aspiration of foreign objects or poisons by children under 4 years.
Caution

Partial or complete absence of lung sounds means *danger.*

A drowsy patient means *danger.*

Status asthmaticus: Acute, severe, or prolonged asthma attack that is not relieved by medication—DANGER
Note

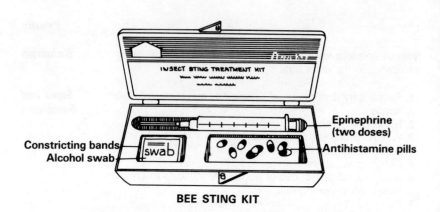

BEE STING KIT

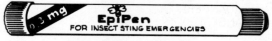

Epinephrine (one dose)

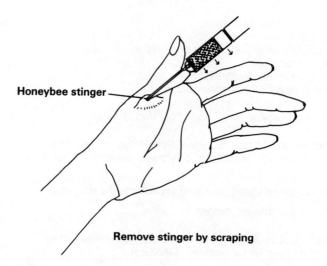

Honeybee stinger

Remove stinger by scraping

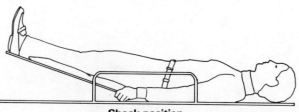

Shock position

Allergic Reaction

1   *Priority*

An acute, potentially life-threatening systemic response to in-   *Definition*
gested, injected, or inhaled foreign substances

1. History of allergic reaction   *Signs and*
2. Respiratory distress, tightness in chest   *Symptoms*
3. Weak, rapid pulse
4. Warm, moist skin
5. Edema (eyelids, lips, tongue, larynx, hands, feet, genitals)
6. Difficulty speaking; barking; high-pitched cough; wheezing; stridor; hoarseness; "lump in throat"
7. Hives, itching
8. Numbness, tingling, prickling
9. Hypotension
10. Nausea, vomiting, diarrhea, abdominal cramps
11. Lightheadedness, dizziness, fainting
12. Apprehension, restlessness
13. Urinary incontinence
14. Headache, unconsciousness

1. Secure and maintain airway   *Treatment*
2. Place patient in shock position
3. Administer O_2 nonbreather
4. Apply constricting band above sting if extremity (follow
   local protocol)
5. Ask for and help patient to administer epinephrine (bee
   sting kit) or antihistamine tablets (follow local protocol)
6. Apply ice pack to sting; MAST (follow local protocol)

Shock position; *rapid;* do *not* delay   *Transport*

Anaphylactic shock is a TRUE EMERGENCY that may develop   *Caution*
rapidly even from a mild allergic reaction.

Symptoms may take up to 24 hours to appear, or may reappear
after initial reaction. Death risk increases with speed symptoms
appear.

Transport hoarseness or stridor patient *at once.*

Remove honeybee stinger if it can be done quickly; scrape   *Note*
away with knife blade; do *not* squeeze.

Angina Pain Characteristics

1. Brought on by exertion or extremes in weather (heat, cold, humidity, wind)
2. Relieved by rest or nitroglycerin
3. Pain feels like pressure or squeezing
4. Pain may radiate to jaw or arms
5. Dyspnea or nausea may accompany pain
6. Pain lasts less than 10 minutes

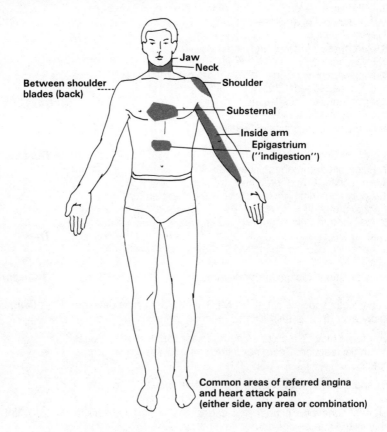

Jaw
Neck
Shoulder
Between shoulder blades (back)
Substernal
Inside arm
Epigastrium ("indigestion")

Common areas of referred angina and heart attack pain (either side, any area or combination)

Angina

1	*Priority*

A sudden attack of periodic chest pain that radiates down the inside of the left arm, often accompanied by feelings of suffocation and impending death — *Definition*

1. Pain: substernal, across chest; radiating to left or both arms, jaw, epigastrium ("squeezing," "aching"); lasts 3–10 minutes; sudden or gradual onset (may start in or be limited to epigastrium, abdominal region, jaw, or back) — *Signs and Symptoms*
2. Apprehension, anxiety
3. Weakness; patient remains still
4. Diaphoresis
5. Shortness of breath
6. Nausea, belching, desire to urinate
7. Previous history of angina

1. Secure and maintain airway — *Treatment*
2. Place patient in semi-reclining position; do *not* let patient move self
3. Administer O_2 (nasal cannula; 4–6 lmp)
4. Loosen restrictive clothing
5. Monitor vital signs
6. Assist with nitroglycerine (follow local protocol)
7. Reassure and keep patient calm
8. Listen to apical beat to detect dysrhythmias

Semi-Fowler's; avoid using siren — *Transport*

Transport even though pain subsides. — *Note*

Do *not* let patient move self; lift and carry.

Pain remains unchanged with breathing and position changes.

Angina may indicate worsening coronary artery disease.

Cannot be differentiated from MI.

See Characteristics on opposite page.

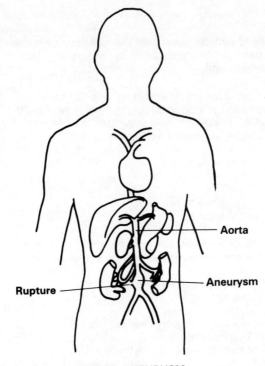

AORTIC ANEURYSM

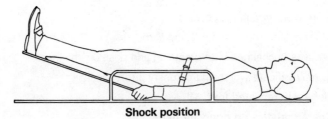

Shock position

Aortic Aneurysm

1	*Priority*

A localized ballooning of the aortic wall | *Definition*

1. History of hypertension or atherosclerosis | *Signs and*
2. History of previous aneurysm | *Symptoms*
3. Severe pain ("tearing"); chest, progressing to legs, back; unchanged with change in position
4. Pulsating mass in abdomen (abdominal aneurysm)
5. Rising blood pressure
6. Fainting (with or without pain)
7. Tachycardia
8. Dyspnea
9. Shock
10. Signs and symptoms of acute abdomen (see p. 159)
11. Blood pressure varies between limbs
12. Absence of one or more peripheral pulses
13. One or both lower extremities cold and pale
14. Signs of CVA (hemiplegia, paraplegia)

1. Administer O_2 | *Treatment*
2. Treat for shock, MAST (follow local protocol)
3. Monitor vital signs frequently
4. Monitor for signs of cardiac tamponade

Shock position | *Transport*

The rupture of an aneurysm is a TRUE EMERGENCY. | *Caution*

Aneurysm development is asymptomatic; signs and symptoms | *Note*
suggest dissection (bleeding between arterial walls) or rupture
(bleeding into body cavity, thoracic or abdominal).

When taking pulses and blood pressure, do both arms separately and compare; also take carotid pulses.

Aortic aneurysm is more common in men than in women, and is more common in elderly patients.

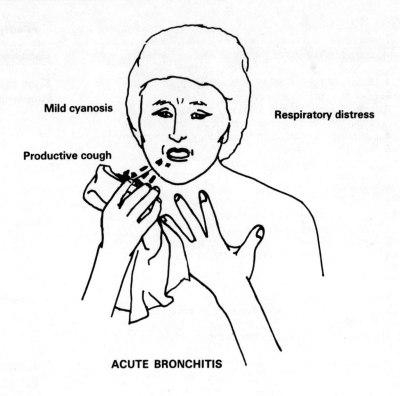

ACUTE BRONCHITIS

Bronchitis (*Acute*)

2 *Priority*

Inflammation of the mucous membranes of the trachea or bron- *Definition*
chus characterized by a frequent, recurring productive cough

1. Respiratory distress, rales, rhonchi, wheezes *Signs and*
2. Productive cough; worsens at night or in damp weather *Symptoms*
3. Mild cyanosis
4. History of inhalation of irritant

1. Secure and maintain airway *Treatment*
2. Administer O_2
3. Have patient sit up

Fowler's; semi-Fowler's *Transport*

Often caused by chronic irritation from smoking or air pollution; *Note*
chronic inhalation of irritating substances; chronic respiratory
tract infections

Common in men middle aged and older.

See also COPD (Emphysema), p. 175.

Common Causes of Coma

Acute infectious disease with encephalitis
Allergic reactions
Body chemistry imbalance
Brain tumor
CVA
Diabetes
Drug or alcohol abuse, suicide attempt
Head trauma
Heat stroke
Hematoma
Hypoglycemia
Hypoxia
Infection or infectious disease
Poisoning
Psychogenic trauma
Reye's syndrome
Shock
Vascular disease

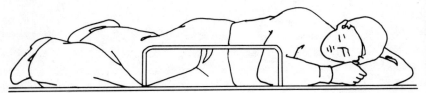

Coma Position

Coma

1

A state of profound unconsciousness from which the patient *Definition*
cannot be aroused

1. Profound unconsciousness *Signs and*
2. Abnormal respiratory patterns, eye signs, reflexes, body *Symptoms*
   movement, posture
3. No response or inappropriate response to stimuli
4. Altered mental state; change in level of consciousness
5. Evidence of drug or alcohol abuse or diabetes

1. Secure and maintain airway; insert airway *Treatment*
2. Treat as spinal injury until proved otherwise
3. Administer O_2; assist ventilations
4. Monitor vital signs (repeat every 5 minutes)
5. Monitor neurological signs (repeat every 15 minutes)
6. Place patient in coma or supine position
7. Monitor for vomiting; be prepared to suction
8. Keep warm
9. Remove contact lenses (follow local protocol)
10. Cover eyes with gauze if no blink reflex
11. Protect from injury

Coma or supine; *rapid* *Transport*

A coma patient often loses protective airway reflexes; monitor *Caution*
breathing; prepare to suction.

Treat coma patient as a spinal injury until ruled out.

A coma patient may see, hear, and understand although unable *Remember*
to respond; treat and reassure accordingly.

Always check for Medic Alert tag on coma patients.

A coma patient is totally dependent on you.

172

Common Causes of Congestive Heart Failure

Bradycardia
Cardiomyopathy (disease of the myocardium)
Coronary artery disease
Drugs
Dysrhythmias
Hypertension
Hyperthyroidism
Intracranial head injury
Myocardial infarction
O_2 toxicity
Uremic poisoning

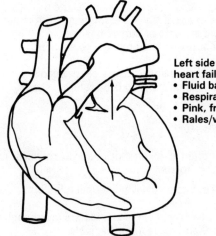

Right side heart failure
• Fluid backs up into extremities
• Neck veins distend
• Edema in extremities, lumbar area, abdomen

Left side heart failure
• Fluid backs up into lungs
• Respiratory distress
• Pink, frothy sputum
• Rales/wheezes

CONGESTIVE HEART FAILURE

173

Congestive Heart Failure (*CHF*)

1 *Priority*

Fluid accumulation in lungs or extremities due to inadequate circulation caused by heart muscle damage (heart disease/MI) — *Definition*

Signs and Symptoms
1. Respiratory distress (left-side CHF)
2. Fatigue, weakness, confusion
3. Cyanosis
4. Diaphoresis
5. Neck vein distension (right-side CHF)
6. Rising blood pressure
7. Pink frothy sputum (left-side CHF)
8. Anxious, restless, combative
9. Rales (bilateral); wheezes
10. Edema—extremities, lumbar, abdomen (right-side CHF)
11. Tachycardia

Treatment
1. Secure and maintain airway
2. Sit patient up, dangle legs (left-side CHF)
3. Administer O_2 as required (100%; demand valve if needed)
4. Monitor vital signs
5. Auscultate lungs; listen for congestion, rales

Fowler's; prompt — *Transport*

A sudden worsening of chronic CHF may indicate MI. — *Caution*

Right or left ventricular failure may occur separately or in combination. — *Remember*

Severe respiratory distress may be a sign of pulmonary edema.

Complication: CO_2 Narcosis (Elevated CO_2 in Blood)

Symptoms include
    Sleepiness
    Restlessness, confusion, agitation, anxiety
    Falling blood pressure
    Flushed face
    Flaccid or twitching muscles
    Congestive heart failure
    Respiratory failure
Treatment
    Secure and maintain airway
    Administer O_2, low level (follow local protocol)
    High Fowler's position
    Transport at once

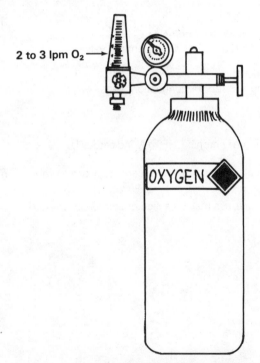

2 to 3 lpm O_2

OXYGEN

**Administer low concentration of oxygen
(follow local protocol)**

COPD (*Chronic Bronchitis/Emphysema*)

1   *Priority*

Inflammation of bronchial tree mucosa with a productive cough   *Definition*
for 3 months in 2 successive years, or pathological changes in
lung tissue with loss of elasticity and gas exchange

1. History of COPD or chronic bronchitis   *Signs and*
2. Respiratory distress, tachypnea, rales, rhonchi, wheezes,   *Symptoms*
   squeaks, lips pursed, breathes in puffs
3. Persistent cough (productive: yellow-green)
4. Barrel chest, unequal expansion
5. Tachycardia, irregular pulse
6. Anxious, restless, confused, weak, sleepy
7. Muscular twitching
8. Fever
9. Thin, wasted look
10. Sits upright and forward
11. Nasal flaring
12. Speaks in short sentences
13. Clubbed fingernails
14. Neck vein distension
15. Lower extremity edema
16. Normal blood pressure
17. Older person

1. Secure and maintain airway   *Treatment*
2. Sit patient up
3. Administer O_2 (1–3 lpm), nasal cannula/24% venturi);
   assist ventilations as required
4. Monitor vital signs
5. Keep warm, avoid overheating
6. Loosen restrictive clothing
7. Monitor breathing and encourage coughing
8. Auscultate lungs

High Fowler's; prompt   *Transport*

High O_2 will *reduce* breathing response; use caution but do *not*   *Caution*
withhold O_2 if in respiratory distress.

Monitor breathing when administering O_2; be prepared to assist ventilations.

Common Causes of Dehydration

Acute alcohol debilitation
Burns
Blood loss
Diabetic crisis
Profuse sweating
Protracted vomiting or diarrhea
Insufficient fluid intake, especially in very young or very old patients

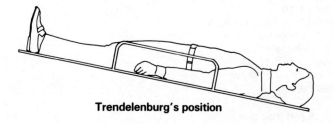

Trendelenburg's position

Dehydration (*Acute Body Fluid Loss*)

1	*Priority*

A 10% or greater loss of total body weight within 24–48 hours — *Definition*

Signs and Symptoms
1. Blood loss; draining wounds
2. Prolonged diarrhea, vomiting, appetite loss
3. Heavy sweating
4. Burns
5. Extreme thirst
6. Dry, cracked mucous membranes; furrows on tongue or sticky tongue
7. Thick, sticky saliva
8. Lax, gray, pale, cool skin
9. Depressed fontanelles (infant)
10. Anxious, irritable, restless
11. Tachycardia
12. Low blood pressure
13. Scant or no urine output
14. Weak muscles, lethargic
15. Abdominal distension
16. Mental dullness; depressed level of consciousness

Treatment
1. Secure and maintain airway
2. Treat for shock
3. Monitor vital signs and level of consciousness

Transport

Shock position

Caution

Shock from rapid dehydration may occur within minutes and is possible with an excessive body fluid loss.

Note

Watch for signs of infection or contagious disease and take necessary precautions against transmission.

178

Common Causes of Diabetic Crises

Insulin Shock (*Hypoglycemia*)
Took too much insulin
Too much exercise
Did not eat enough food
All of the above or in combination
Vomited after taking insulin
Severe emotional stress
Exposure to severe cold

Diabetic Coma
Failed to take insulin/medication
Ate too much
Severe infection or stress
Dehydration, vomiting

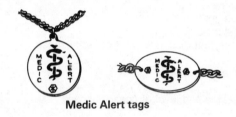

Medic Alert tags

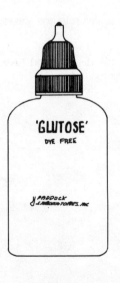

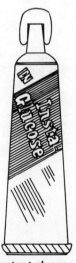

Instant glucose

Diabetes (*Diabetic Coma/Insulin Shock*)

1   *Priority*

A potentially life-threatening metabolic disorder involving insulin production and sugar utilization   *Definition*

INSULIN SHOCK (Hypoglycemia)	DIABETIC COMA (Hyperglycemia)
1. Rapid onset	1. Gradual onset
2. Too much insulin; too little food; too much exercise	2. Too little insulin; too much food
3. Shallow breathing	3. Rapid, deep breathing
4. Pale, cool, moist skin, profuse perspiration	4. Warm, dry skin; fever
5. Full, rapid pulse	5. Weak, rapid pulse
6. Normal blood pressure	6. Low BP on standing
7. Intense hunger	7. Abdominal pain, nausea, vomiting, dehydration
8. Dizziness, tremors	8. Sweet, fruity breath
9. Headache, double vision	9. Intense thirst, red lips
10. Apathy, irritability	10. Frequent urination
11. Fainting, seizure, coma	11. Dim vision, sunken eyes
	12. Unconsciousness

Signs and Symptoms

ASK: Did you eat today/take your insulin today?   *Treatment*

CONSCIOUS	CONSCIOUS
1. Administer sugar by mouth	1. Shock position
2. Monitor vital signs	2. Administer O_2
3. Keep warm (blanket)	3. Keep warm (blanket)
	4. Immediate transport

UNCONSCIOUS (Insulin Shock/Diabetic Coma)
1. Assure and maintain airway
2. Administer O_2
3. Coma position (feet elevated)
4. Keep warm (blanket)

Unconscious, coma position; conscious, shock position   *Transport*

Do *not* administer liquids to unconscious patient.   *Caution*

If in doubt between insulin shock or diabetic coma, administer sugar: glucose, fruit juice, candy, corn syrup, honey, etc.   *Note*

If patient's blood sugar level is determined by a home glucose monitor, call medical control with results and for advice.   *Special Consideration*

Assessing Pain

1. Establish previous history of similar pain
2. Have patient relate and compare pain characteristics
   a. Quality
   b. Quantity
   c. Location of primary and referred sites
   d. Duration
   e. What initiates the pain?
   f. What aggravates the pain?
   g. What alleviates the pain?
   h. What past treatment has he had? Was it effective?

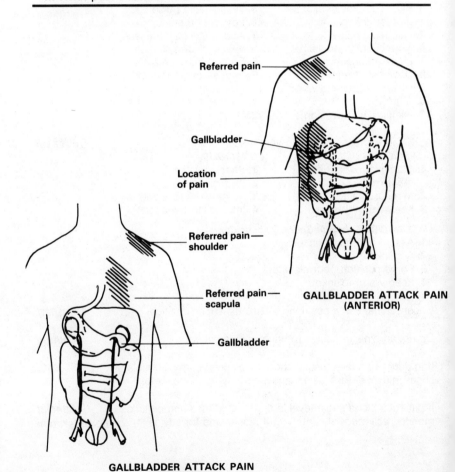

GALLBLADDER ATTACK PAIN
(ANTERIOR)

GALLBLADDER ATTACK PAIN
(POSTERIOR)

Gallbladder Attack

2   *Priority*

Acute inflammation of the gallbladder usually caused by gall-stone obstructing bile duct   *Definition*

1. History of previous attacks   *Signs and*
2. Slow onset of dull epigastric pain   *Symptoms*
3. Pain, sharp, RUQ; referred pain, right scapula or shoulder
4. Nausea, vomiting, diaphoresis
5. Fever
6. Jaundice

1. Obtain history of pain   *Treatment*
2. Administer O_2 if anxious or if respiratory distress
3. Keep warm; reassure
4. Monitor vital signs
5. Rule out heart attack
6. Nothing by mouth

Position of comfort   *Transport*

Pain may suggest heart attack; rule out MI.   *Caution*

Be alert for signs and complications of peritonitis.

Signs and symptoms of peritonitis
1. Localized or diffuse abdominal pain
2. Movement intensifies pain
3. Rising temperature
4. Increased heart rate
5. Chills

Common Causes and Sources of GI Bleeding

Alcohol abuse
Aspirin (excessive use)
Cancer
Cecal ulcers
Diverticulitis
Duodenal ulcers
Esophageal varices
Gastritis
Hemorrhoids
Intestinal irritation (food allergy)
Peptic ulcer
Polyps

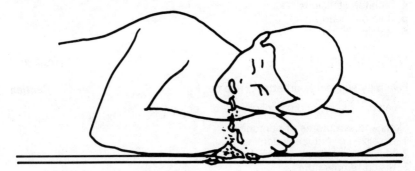

**Check vomitus for blood
(save specimen)**

Gastrointestinal Bleeding

1   *Priority*

Any bleeding in the gastrointestinal tract, from mouth to anus   *Definition*

1. Blood in sputum, vomitus (coffee ground), or stool (tarry);   *Signs and*
   rectal bleeding   *Symptoms*
2. Abdominal pain, cramps, tenderness, fluid, distension
3. Weakness; fainting (if heavy blood loss)
4. Pallor; jaundice (if liver disease)
5. Tachycardia
6. Falling blood pressure, rising pulse
7. Rising respirations
8. Fever

1. Secure and maintain airway   *Treatment*
2. Administer O_2
3. Treat for shock; MAST if indicated
4. Monitor vital signs and level of consciousness
5. Anticipate vomiting; prepare to suction
6. Give nothing by mouth

Position of comfort; shock position   *Transport*

GI bleeding is a symptom of an underlying condition and must   *Caution*
be evaluated by a physician.

GI bleeding may have sudden onset or may occur over a long   *Note*
period.

Save stool or vomitus specimen for ER evaluation.

Hemoptysis (coughing or spitting up blood) may masquerade as
GI bleeding, and vice versa.

Conditions Commonly Related to Headache

Allergies
Brain tumor
Cerebral aneurysm
Cerebral hemorrhage
CO (carbon monoxide) poisoning
CVA (stroke)
Hypertension
Hypoglycemia
Meningitis
Migraine headache
Preeclampsia (toxemia of pregnancy)
Seizures
Sinus infections, congestion
Toxic fume inhalation

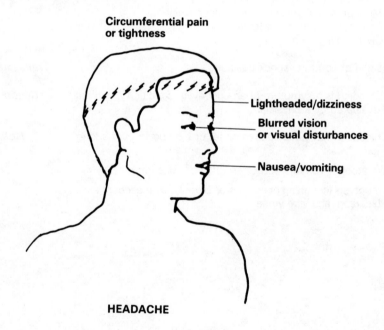

Circumferential pain
or tightness

Lightheaded/dizziness

Blurred vision
or visual disturbances

Nausea/vomiting

HEADACHE

Headache

1, 2, 3 (determined by cause)	*Priority*
The gradual or sudden onset of head pain	*Definition*

1. Mild to severe head pain
2. Blurred vision or vision disturbances
3. Vertigo
4. Nausea, vomiting
5. Tender spots or tightness around head

Signs and Symptoms

1. Reduce noise, dim bright lights
2. Ice pack to head
3. Administer O_2 (nasal cannula)
4. Assess vital signs
5. Monitor level of consciousness; observe changes
6. Rest and relaxation

Treatment

Position of comfort; dim lights

Transport

Headache is often a symptom of an underlying condition. It is essential to rule out or identify all possible causes that may be an immediate threat to life or health. Therefore, determine

Special Attention

1. Patient history
2. Headache history
    a. Duration
    b. Location
    c. Frequency
    d. Time of onset
    e. Mode of onset
    f. Pain quality
3. Precipitating factors
4. Related symptoms
5. Relieving factors

Predisposing Conditions to MI

Family history of MI or heart conditions
Smoking
Elevated cholesterol and serum triglyceride levels
Diabetes
Hypertension
Obese; high fat, carbohydrate, salt intake
Inactive or limited exercise
Complications of aging
Stress, Type A personality (aggressive, workaholic, competitive, impatient)
Male (female incidence rising with smoking, oral contraception, high-stress jobs, postmenopause)

Complications of MI

Cardiac arrest (within 1 hour)
    Treat: CPR
Cardiogenic shock (within 24 hours)
    Treat: Lie patient supine; administer 100% O_2; apply MAST (follow local protocol)
Congestive heart failure
    Treat: Sit patient with legs dangling; administer 100% O_2 unless COPD, then 24%
Pulmonary edema (within 3–7 days)
    Treat: Position of comfort; administer high concentration O_2; assist ventilations as required

Heart Attack (*Myocardial Infarction* [*MI*])

1	**Priority**

The reduction or cessation of circulation through a coronary artery from an embolus, atherosclerosis, or thrombus resulting in heart muscle death — **Definition**

Signs and Symptoms

1. Chest pain (substernal, crushing, squeezing); may radiate to left arm, shoulder blade, neck, jaw, epigastrum; may resemble indigestion; start in epigastric/abdominal region; last longer than 15 minutes, unrelieved by nitroglycerine, rest, antacid
2. Respiratory distress (shallow or deep breaths); coughing (with or without sputum)
3. Sweating; cold, clammy skin; gray pallor; cyanosis
4. Nausea, vomiting, loss of appetite
5. Weakness, fatigue, dizziness
6. Anxious; feels impending doom; depressed; restless; frightened appearance; irritable; fainting
7. Rapid, irregular pulse; low blood pressure
8. Sudden death

Treatment

CONSCIOUS
1. Place in semireclining position; loosen clothing
2. Secure and maintain airway
3. Administer O_2 (6 lpm, nasal cannula; mask if condition worsens)
4. Monitor vital signs, chest sounds, level of consciousness
5. Keep patient calm, warm, reassured
6. Assist with prescribed medications or nitroglycerine (follow local protocol)

UNCONSCIOUS
1. Secure and maintain airway
2. Administer O_2 (high concentration, nonrebreather)
3. Begin CPR if required with bag valve mask or demand valve

Fowler's, semi-Fowler's; *rapid; no* siren — **Transport**

Do *not* let patient exert self; keep patient still; carry patient to cot and ambulance; continue reassurance. — **Caution**

Treat *any adult* with chest pain and *any elderly patient* with sudden weakness, confusion, dyspnea as MI. — **Note**

Explain to patient what you are doing and why.

Frequent Causes of Hypertensive Crisis

Acute left ventricular failure
Eclampsia (grave toxemia of pregnancy)
Intracerebral hemorrhage
MAO inhibitor interactions (antidepressant drugs)
Myocardial ischemia (decreased blood supply)
Renal function abnormality

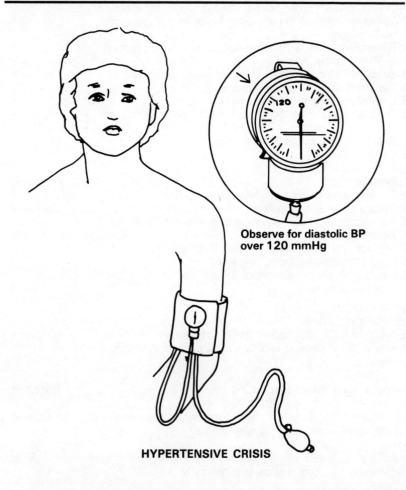

**Observe for diastolic BP
over 120 mmHg**

HYPERTENSIVE CRISIS

Hypertensive Crisis

Priority

A sudden, severe life-threatening rise in blood pressure   *Definition*

Signs and
Symptoms

1. Severe headache
2. Diastolic BP over 120 (as high as 140–150)
3. Drowsiness, confusion, stupor, irritability
4. Blurred vision; double vision
5. Chest pain
6. Ringing in ears
7. Shortness of breath
8. Nausea, vomiting
9. Tachycardia
10. Distended neck veins
11. Nosebleed
12. Twitching muscles
13. Coughing up blood

1. Calm patient; alleviate anxiety   *Treatment*
2. Monitor vital signs; take BP every 5 minutes
3. Administer O_2 (nasal cannula)
4. Monitor level of consciousness

Position of comfort; semi-Fowler's; rapid   *Transport*

Immediate, vigorous medical treatment to lower blood pres-   *Caution*
sure is essential.

Common Causes of Hyperventilation Syndrome

Airway obstruction (partial)
Anxiety, panic, stress
Congestive heart failure (early)
COPD
Diabetic condition (ketoacidosis)
Drug use
Psychogenic (overbreathing, rapid breathing)
Shock

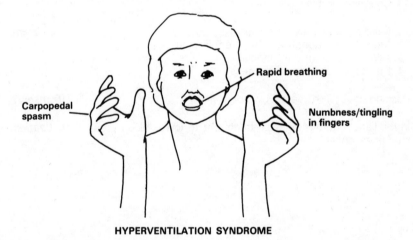

Carpopedal spasm

Rapid breathing

Numbness/tingling in fingers

HYPERVENTILATION SYNDROME

Hyperventilation Syndrome

---

2 *Priority*

A collection of symptoms caused by an abrupt lowering of *Definition*
blood CO_2 level resulting from abnormally deep or rapid breathing, often caused by psychological stress

Three or more of the following may suggest hyperventilation *Signs and*
syndrome: *Symptoms*
1. Strange, hard-to-describe feeling in top of head
2. Dizziness, lightheadedness
3. Blurred vision
4. Mouth dry, bitter
5. Tingling hands, feet, around mouth
6. Tight throat or lump in throat
7. Shortness of breath, rapid breathing
8. Extreme weakness
9. Sense of impending doom
10. Sense of being in a dream
11. Chest pain
12. Contraction of the hands and feet (carpopedal spasm)
13. Rapid heart rate, "pounding" heart

1. Determine if patient is diabetic *Treatment*
2. Calm and reassure patient
3. Help patient reduce respirations by counting aloud 5 seconds between breaths (count: "one thousand one . . .
   one thousand two" . . . etc.)
4. Have patient rebreathe exhaled air from paper bag; do
   not do this if hyperventilation has medical, nonanxiety
   basis
5. Administer O_2 if respiratory distress is from a medical
   condition
6. Explain cause of syndrome after attack
7. Transport for follow up

High Fowler's *Transport*

Cyanosis usually suggests severe respiratory distress, not hy- *Note*
perventilation; therefore, look for a more serious condition if
patient is cyanotic.

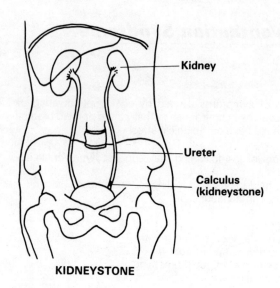

KIDNEYSTONE

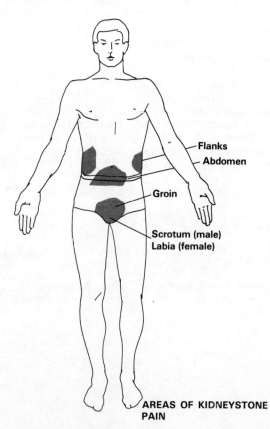

AREAS OF KIDNEYSTONE PAIN

Kidney Stones

Stones or sediment in the urinary system that obstructs the excretion of urine   *Definition*

Signs and Symptoms

1. Intense pain in flank, abdomen, groin (may radiate to scrotum or labia)
2. Distended abdomen
3. Inability to find a comfortable position
4. Sweating, pallor
5. Fever, chills
6. Sense of full bladder; urge to urinate
7. Blood in urine
8. Nausea, vomiting
9. Tachycardia
10. Hypotension
11. Sudden block of urine stream

Treatment

1. Place patient in most comfortable position
2. Monitor vital signs
3. Monitor bladder distension
4. Keep warm
5. Nothing by mouth

Transport

Position of comfort

Note

Observe for blood, stones, or sediment in urine; save urine sample for ER evaluation.

Common Causes of Nosebleed

Bleeding diseases
Dryness of nasal membranes
Exertion
Facial trauma
Head cold
High altitude exposure
Infection
Sinus conditions
Skull fracture
Hypertension

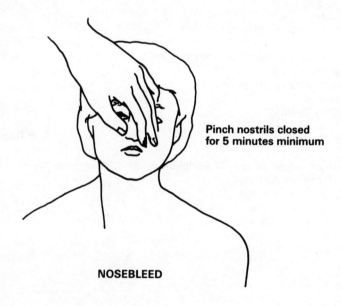

Pinch nostrils closed
for 5 minutes minimum

NOSEBLEED

Nosebleed (*Epistaxis*)

1 or 2 (determined by severity) — ***Priority***

Minor to severe bleeding from the nose — ***Definition***

Signs and Symptoms
1. Bleeding from nose or down throat
2. Anxiety
3. Shock (if massive blood loss)

Treatment
1. Keep patient sitting unless shock is evident
2. Keep patient quiet; have him lean forward over emesis basin
3. Have patient breathe through mouth
4. Pinch nostrils closed for 5 minutes minimum (do *not* do this if nasal fracture)
5. Do *not* block nosebleed if head injury
6. Place rolled dressing under patient's upper lip
7. Place ice pack over nose
8. Be prepared to suction; allow patient to cough or spit up blood
9. Monitor for shock
10. Administer O$_2$ if required

High Fowler's — ***Transport***

Do *not* attempt to stop nosebleed if head injury. — ***Caution***

Nosebleed may be accompanied by respiratory distress, nausea, and vertigo, and may lead to fainting.

Swallowing blood can cause nausea and vomiting; be prepared to suction.

Do *not* pack nostrils. — ***Note***

Visible flow may represent only a small portion; the rest may be swallowed. — ***Remember***

Continue to hold pressure on patient's nostrils if bleeding has not stopped in 5–10 minutes (the normal clotting time for blood).

Common Causes of Pneumonia

Cardiovascular disease
Diabetic conditions
Influenza complications
Poor health; poor general condition
Pulmonary disorders
Smoking
Steroid use
Sudden temperature changes
Vomitus aspiration (especially with alcohol or drug abuse)

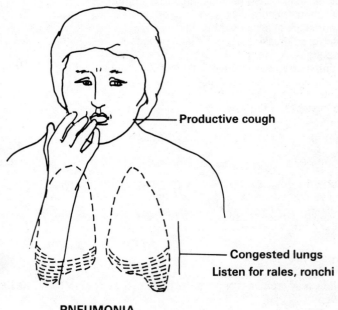

Productive cough

Congested lungs
Listen for rales, ronchi

PNEUMONIA

Acute lung inflammation or filling of alveoli with fluid as a result   *Definition*
of bacterial infection, inspiration of vomitus or liquid, inhalation
of toxic substances, or cancer

Signs and Symptoms

1. Sudden onset
2. Acute respiratory distress; cyanosis
3. High fever (103°F–104°F), chills, muscle aches
4. Dry, hot skin
5. Rapid heartbeat
6. Rales, rhonchi, lung congestion
7. Productive (purulent) cough
8. Chest or abdominal pain
9. Abdominal distension, nausea, vomiting
10. Apprehension

Treatment

1. Assure and maintain airway
2. Assist breathing; administer O_2 (nasal cannula, mask)
3. Monitor vital signs (take temperature)
4. Keep warm
5. Auscultate lungs with stethoscope

Transport

Position of comfort

Note

Use precautions to avoid contamination; use facial mask, rubber gloves; disinfect ambulance after run.

Often occurs in very young patients or very old patients in weakened condition.

Predisposing Factors for Pulmonary Embolism

Acute infections
Air emboli
Blood diseases
Cardiac diseases
Childbirth
Congenital heart failure
Long bone fracture
Neoplasms (abnormal new tissue growth)
Obesity
Oral contraceptives
Prolonged bed rest and long trips
Surgery
Thrombophlebitis
Trauma

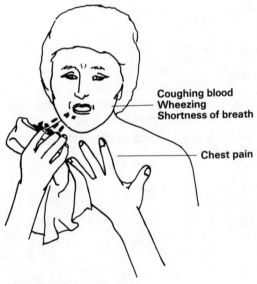

Coughing blood
Wheezing
Shortness of breath

Chest pain

PULMONARY EMBOLISM

Pulmonary Embolism

1   *Priority*

The obstruction of a pulmonary artery by a foreign substance   *Definition*
such as air, fat, tissue, or blood clot

1. Sudden chest pain, increases with deep breath   *Signs and*
2. Respiratory distress, shortness of breath   *Symptoms*
3. Rising pulse; falling blood pressure
4. Wheezing
5. Coughing up blood
6. Cyanosis, pallor
7. Anxiety
8. Shock
9. Lower leg vein inflammation

1. Assure and maintain airway   *Treatment*
2. Assist breathing; administer O_2 (high concentration, nonrebreather)
3. Monitor vitals
4. Treat for shock if indicated
5. Observe for pulmonary edema
6. Auscultate lungs with stethoscope

Position of comfort; determined by patient's condition   *Transport*

Pulmonary embolism is difficult to distinguish from pneumonia,   *Note*
MI, or pneumothorax.

Common Causes of Seizure

Age related, in elderly patient
Alcohol or drug abuse, withdrawal
Birth injury
Brain tumor or injury
Cerebral embolus
Disease, illness, infection
Epilepsy
Extreme stress
High fever
Large intake of caffeine
Medication overdose

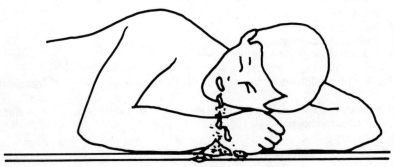

Seizure Transport

- Coma position
- Observe for frothy mucus
- Prepare to suction

Seizure (*Convulsion*)

1 *Priority*

A sudden episode of disturbed brain cell electrical activity, often with involuntary muscle activity, changes in sensation, behavior, level of consciousness, and loss of consciousness *Definition*

Signs and Symptoms

1. Patient reports pre-seizure sensation of light (aura), color, or smell.
2. Sudden loss of consciousness
3. Short period of muscle stiffening
4. Incontinence of bowel or bladder
5. Difficult, rapid breathing; cyanosis
6. Jaw muscle contraction; biting of tongue, lips
7. Drooling, foaming at mouth
8. Disorientation
9. Diaphoresis, cyanosis during seizure
10. Tachycardia

Treatment

1. Secure and maintain airway; be prepared to suction
2. Look for other injuries
3. Administer O_2 by mask (high concentration if status epilepticus)
4. Assist ventilations as required if status epilepticus
5. Do not restrain
6. Protect from injury
7. Loosen restrictive clothing; keep warm
8. Monitor vital signs and pupils
9. Monitor for *status epilepticus*
10. Place in coma position after seizure

Coma position; suction; *rapid* for status epilepticus *Transport*

Do *not* force fingers or items into mouth during seizure. *Caution*

Status epilepticus: additional seizures without gaining full consciousness between seizures; A TRUE EMERGENCY.

Grand mal, full body convulsion; *petit mal,* brief loss of awareness *Note*

Common Causes of Spontaneous Pneumothorax

Assisted ventilation (positive pressure)
Cancer
Chest compression
Emphysema
Spontaneous from areas on lung surfaces (ruptures) (especially in young, thin adults)
Tuberculosis
Trauma

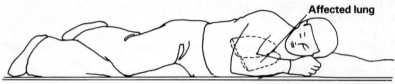

Affected lung

Affected Side Transport Position

Spontaneous Pneumothorax

1   *Priority*

Sudden lung collapse due to the rupture of a weak area on the   *Definition*
lung surface

1. Sudden, sharp unilateral chest or shoulder pain   *Signs and*
2. Decreasing breath sounds; increasing respirations   *Symptoms*
3. Extreme anxiety, agitation
4. Coughing
5. May progress to tension pneumothorax
   a. Mediastinal/tracheal shift to unaffected side
   b. Distended neck veins
   c. Hollow affected side chest sounds
   d. Shock
   e. Cyanosis

1. Secure and maintain airway   *Treatment*
2. Assist breathing; high concentration O_2
3. Monitor vital signs
4. Observe for tension pneumothorax

Semi-Fowler's or affected side down   *Transport*

Monitor for tension pneumothorax.   *Caution*

Occurs more frequently in men than in women and older pa-   *Note*
tients with COPD, but can occur in healthy young adults.

Factors Increasing Risk of Stroke

Arrhythmias
Cardiac/myocardial enlargement
Diabetes mellitus
Family history of CVA
Gout
High levels of serum triglycerides
Hypertension
Hypotension on standing
Lack of exercise
Oral contraceptive use
Rheumatic heart disease
Smoking
TIAs

Transient Ischemic Attack (TIA) Syndrome

Signs and Symptoms
1. Headache, blurry vision one or both eyes, partial or temporary loss of vision
2. Lightheadedness, dizziness, fainting (syncope)
3. Confusion; speech or memory impairment; sensory disturbances
4. Loss of muscle tone in extremities
5. Seizure

Treatment
1. Secure and maintain airway
2. Administer O_2
3. Monitor vital signs
4. Reassure

Transport
Position of comfort; coma if unconscious

Warning TIA may mean an impending CVA; transport all TIA patients for evaluation

Stroke (*Cerebrovascular Accident [CVA]*)

1   *Priority*

The sudden impairment by embolism or hemorrhage of the   *Definition*
blood vessels supplying the brain, resulting in damage from
reduced brain tissue oxygenation

1. Headache, confusion, decreased consciousness (dizziness   *Signs and*
   to coma)   *Symptoms*
2. Temporary weakness or paralysis of face, arms, legs
3. Hemiplegia (one-sided paralysis/loss of function)
4. Facial flaccidity, loss of expression, flushed, pale
5. Speech defects (speaking, comprehension)
6. Vision defects (loss/dimness, especially one eye; double
   vision)
7. Personality change; decrease in mental ability; inability to
   concentrate
8. Hypertension
9. Unequal pupil size
10. Rapid, strong pulse
11. Respiratory distress
12. Convulsions
13. Nausea
14. Loss of bowel and bladder control

1. Secure and maintain airway; remove dentures   *Treatment*
2. Administer O_2 (nasal cannula); assist ventilations if
   needed
3. Monitor vital signs (radial *and* carotid pulses)
4. Keep warm and quiet; reassure
5. Protect paralyzed extremities, especially when moving
6. Avoid unnecessary movement
7. Nothing by mouth
8. Monitor level of consciousness
9. Be prepared to suction

Lateral recumbent (coma position) with affected limbs beneath   *Transport*
patient; avoid rough handling

High BP with falling pulse: transport immediately.   *Caution*

An unconscious patient may be able to hear you; say nothing   *Note*
that would increase anxiety.

Treat stroke patients with tender loving care.

This section reviews common environmental emergencies in alphabetical order.

Guidelines

1. Remove any risk of personal injury before proceeding.
2. Complete surveys and histories are required for proper care.
3. **Signs and Symptoms** listed here include most but not necessarily all the signs and symptoms for a given emergency.
4. In general, the order of signs and symptoms is high to low priority, most to least evident, and most to least common.
5. In general, signs and symptoms are grouped by relationship to a common organ, function, or other shared characteristic.
6. The presence of a sign or symptom and *not* its place on the list determines its significance in assessing a condition.
7. All, some, or no signs and symptoms may be present; they are intended only to aid patient assessment and may suggest a condition that requires evaluation by a physician.
8. **Treatment** described here refers only to minimum suggested approved procedures for use by qualified personnel, generally from most important to least important.
9. All injuries and medical conditions must be individually assessed and treated according to local standards and protocols.

This section will help you to

1. Identify, assess, and treat the named conditions.
2. Prepare for transport and transport affected patients.

Special Considerations

Request police/rabies control officer assistance to
    a. Identify animal/fish
    b. Assess its behavior
    c. Capture or kill for transport if required
Do *not* risk personal injury
Complications may include
    a. Rabies
    b. Infection
    c. Anaphylactic shock
Apply tourniquets above and below stings
    a. Follow local protocol
    b. Restrict venous flow only, *NOT* arterial flow

Types

BITES
Animal

Dog	Skunk	Hamster
Cat	Squirrel	Wolf
Bat	Raccoon	Bear
Fox	Gerbil	Human

Sea Animal

Shark	Sea snake	Sea lion
Barracuda	Octopus	Seal
Moray eel	Squid	Killer whale

STINGS
Insects   *Sea animal*

Bee	Spider	Jellyfish
Wasp	Scorpion	Portuguese man-of-war
Hornet		Anemone
		Coral

SPINES
Sea Animal

Stingray	Catfish
Sea urchin	Scorpion fish

Caution

Sea animal venom may be discharged by mechanical or chemical stimulation.

Tentacles of dead animal may continue to discharge venom; can contaminate patient, others.

Reactions to venoms may be instant or delayed.

Human bites can be infectious; determine patient's last tetanus injection and biter's history of communicable disease.

Determine animal bite victim's last tetanus injection, animal's health, and health history if possible.

Bites (Animal/Sea Animal/Human)

Determined by severity	**Priority**
Broken or punctured skin caused by the teeth or spines of land or sea animals	**Definition**

ANIMAL/HUMAN BITES
1. Visible wounds, bleeding, teeth marks
2. Redness, swelling, bruising, warmth at site
3. Infection, pus, foul-smelling gray secretion

Signs and Symptoms

1. Treat serious and life-threatening injuries
2. Cleanse wound with soap and water; alcohol rinse
3. Dress, bandage, immobilize

Treatment

SEA ANIMAL STINGS
1. Visible punctures, sting marks
2. Pain, redness, swelling, numbness at site
3. Faintness, weakness; shock
4. Chills, fever

Signs and Symptoms

1. Rinse wounds with alcohol
2. Apply baking soda solution
3. Apply meat tenderizer if possible, or dry powder
4. Scrape off nematocysts ("stingers") with knife; remove spines
5. Rinse with baking soda solution
6. Apply cold pack to area
7. Treat related conditions
8. Monitor vital signs
9. Observe for anaphylactic or allergic reactions
10. Contact ER physician if uncertain

Treatment

POISONOUS FISH/SHELLFISH
1. Headache, muscle pain, pain at site
2. Respiratory distress, laryngeal edema
3. Nausea, vomiting
4. Burning, tingling lips, face, tongue
5. Intense thirst, weakness, salivation, paralysis

Signs and Symptoms

1. Secure and maintain airway
2. Monitor vital signs, breathing changes, hoarseness, stridor
3. Transport at once

Treatment

Position of comfort; shock position; elevate extremities

Transport

Treatment
1. Secure and maintain airway
2. Administer O_2 (high concentration, humidified) as required
3. Immerse burned area in cool water or cover with wet burn sheet or dressing; *avoid* overcooling
4. Cover burn with burn sheet
   a. If eyes: keep closed; cover with sterile pads.
      Note: thermal burn only; *not* chemical burn
   b. Separate fingers/toes with moist, sterile pads
5. Treat for shock; apply MAST (follow local protocol)
6. Transport in position of comfort; elevate extremities; cover with sterile burn sheets; avoid overcooling

Rule of Nines *TO ESTIMATE BURNED AREA*

Adult

Head and neck,	9%
Anterior trunk,	18%
(Thorax,	9%)
(Abdomen,	9%)
Posterior trunk,	18%
(Upper back,	9%)
(Lower back,	9%)
Upper extremities,	9% each
Lower extremities,	18% each
Genital area,	1%

Infant/Child
Use same percentages
as adult except:
Head, 18%
Legs, 14%

High-Risk Patients

Infants, children under 5 years
Elderly
Diabetic
Heart or major disease
Related injuries

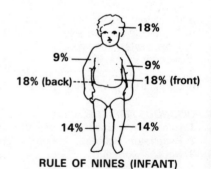

9% ―
18% (back)―
18%
9%
18% (front)
14% ― ― 14%

RULE OF NINES (INFANT)

Burn Assessment

1, 2 (determined by severity)	*Priority*

1ST DEGREE
1. Redness, pain, tenderness
2. Blanching on pressure
3. Edema
4. Epidermis damage only

3RD DEGREE
1. Leathery, charred, pearly gray skin
2. No pain or sensitivity
3. No blanching
4. Epidermis, dermis

Definition

2ND DEGREE
1. Redness, mottling, pain
2. Blistering
3. Blanching on pressure
4. Epidermis, part of dermis damaged

4TH DEGREE
1. Damage through muscle, bone; entrance and exit wound

Severity	Degree	Body Area (%)	Complication	Assessment
Minor	1, 2, 3	Minimal	None	
Moderate	2	Adult, 15–20 Child, 10–20	None	
	3	All ages, 2–10		
Major	2	Adult, 25+ Child, 20+	Face, eye, ear, hand, crotch burns; in-	
	3	All ages, 10+	halation injuries; fracture, trauma; infant, elderly	

Thermal: contact with flame, hot gases, hot object
Electrical: contact with electric current, lightning
Chemical: contact with strong acid, alkali
Inhalation: inhalation of heat, smoke, noxious gases, chemical

Categories

See Definition above.

Signs and Symptoms

See facing page.

Treatment

Position of comfort, determined by complications

Transport

Burns may be a combination of 1st, 2nd, and 3rd degree.

Remember

Special Cases

HYDROFLUORIC ACID
1. Flush burned area with copious amounts of cool water for minimum 10 minutes
2. Remove all contaminated clothing
3. Administer 100% humidified O_2

DRY LIME
1. Brush away as much as possible *before* flushing
2. Remove all contaminated articles of clothing
3. Flush rapidly, thoroughly, continuously

CARBOLIC ACID (Phenol)
1. Rinse with alcohol if possible before flushing with water (do *not* put alcohol in eyes)

SULFURIC ACID
1. First rinse with soapy water solution, followed by steady flushing with tepid water

LYE
1. Do *not* induce vomiting if swallowed
2. Flush with copious amounts of water if external

Remember

No high pressure when flushing; use full, steady stream.

When only one eye is affected, place patient on side with that eye down so rinse will not reach unaffected eye.

Use only tepid *water* to flush or irrigate eyes and tissues; do not use neutralizers.

Contact medical control for advice and treatment.

Chemical Burns

1, 2, 3 (determined by severity)

Tissue injury caused by exposure to strong acid or alkali   *Definition*

Signs and symptoms vary with chemical causing injury and area   *Signs and*
of injury. They may include   *Symptoms*
1. Visible injured or irritated tissue (skin, eyes, mucous membranes)
2. Visible chemical residue on tissue or clothing
3. Visible or smelly fumes at scene or on patient
4. Respiratory distress
5. Unconsciousness

Initiate treatment *immediately.*   *Treatment*

BODY SURFACE
1. Begin flushing burned area with a full but gentle steady
   stream of tepid *water* (hose, shower) at *once*
   a. Do *not* waste time removing clothes
   b. Do *not* waste time looking for antidote
2. Remove clothing and continue to flush until chemical is
   removed (at least 5–10 minutes)
3. Cover burns with dry, sterile dressings

EYES
1. Flush *immediately* with steady stream of *water* with head
   turned sideways if patient supine
2. Remove contact lenses
3. Flush under eyelids
4. Continue to irrigate until chemical is removed
   a. Minimum 20 minutes; 30 if an alkali
5. Do *not* apply chemical antidote to eyes
6. Do *not* let patient rub eyes
7. Close and cover eyes with loose, sterile dressing after
   flushing for at least 30 minutes

Position of comfort; continue to flush affected area en route   *Transport*

See Special Cases on facing page   *Note*

Lightning Injury Complications

Nervous system impairment, unconsciousness
Sensory deprivation: hearing, sight, speech
Cardiovascular effects: dysrrhythmias, loss of pulse, cardiac arrest
Burns, traumatic injury
Respiratory center paralysis (respiratory arrest)

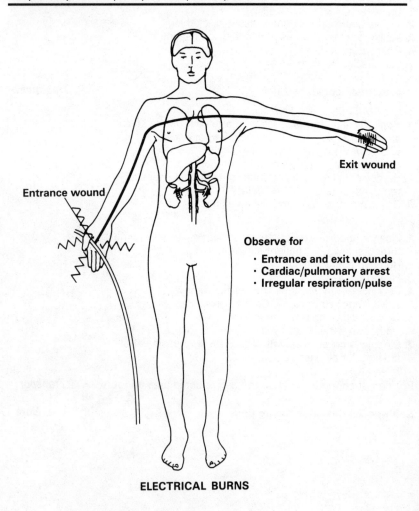

Exit wound

Entrance wound

Observe for

· **Entrance and exit wounds**
· **Cardiac/pulmonary arrest**
· **Irregular respiration/pulse**

ELECTRICAL BURNS

Electrical/Lightning Burns

Tissue damage resulting from contact with electric current or   *Definition*
lightning

ELECTROCUTION/LIGHTNING   *Signs and*
1. Visible tissue damage (entry and exit wound)   *Symptoms*
2. Dazed, confused
3. Weak, irregular or no pulse
4. Shallow, irregular or no breathing
5. Fractures

1. Remove patient from electrical contact   *Treatment*
   a. Avoid risk of personal injury
2. Secure and maintain airway; *immediate* CPR if indicated
   a. Do *not* hyperextend lightning victim's neck
3. Administer O_2; assist breathing
4. Survey; treat for burns, entrance *and* exit wounds, tissue
   damage, fractures
   a. Treat lightning victim as spinal injury
   b. Cool electrical burns with cool water, moist dressing;
      cover with moist dressing
5. Monitor vital signs and breathing
6. Treat for shock
7. Prepare to suction unconscious patient

Conscious, semi-Fowler's; unconscious, coma   *Transport*

Respiratory and cardiac arrest are the major concerns in electro- *Caution*
cution and lightning victims.

Do *not* risk personal injury. Make certain victim and area are
safe before acting. Defer to rescue, fire, or power company
personnel.

Vehicles, guard rails, and metal fences are conductors.   *Remember*

When more than one person is struck by lightning, treat the
apparently dead *first*; those with vital signs should recover
spontaneously; treat all burns.

Special Treatment

1ST AND 2ND DEGREE BURNS
1. Place affected limb in cold water; wrap affected part in cool, moist sheet
2. Avoid overcooling

EYE BURNS
1. Do *not* open burned lids
2. Make sure burn is not chemical
   a. If it is, irrigate, flush chemicals
3. Cover *both* eyes with moist, sterile pads

HAND OR FOOT BURNS
1. Separate fingers/toes with sterile, moist pads or non-adherent dressings

SUNBURN
1. If 1st degree, apply cool, moist dressing
2. If 2nd degree, treat as above and transport

SCALDS
1. Treat as thermal burn

RESPIRATORY TRACT (Burns, Smoke Inhalation)
1. Secure and maintain airway
2. Administer O_2 (high concentration, nonrebreather)
3. Treat for shock
4. Monitor vital signs
5. *Rapid* transport; shock position if shock

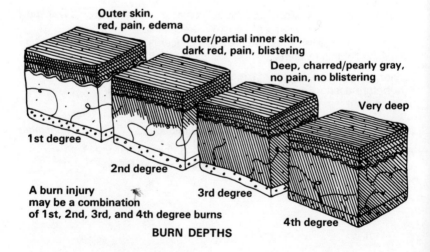

Outer skin, red, pain, edema

Outer/partial inner skin, dark red, pain, blistering

Deep, charred/pearly gray, no pain, no blistering

Very deep

1st degree

2nd degree

3rd degree

4th degree

A burn injury may be a combination of 1st, 2nd, 3rd, and 4th degree burns

BURN DEPTHS

Thermal Burns

1, 2   *Priority*

Tissue damage resulting from exposure to heat or flame   *Definition*

See also Burn Assessment p. 210, 211   *Assessment*
1st Degree: outer skin, red, pain, edema
2nd Degree: outer/partial inner skin, dark red, pain, blistering
3rd Degree: deep, charred/pearly gray, no pain, no blistering
4th Degree: very deep, very charred, loss of function, no pain

1. Obvious tissue damage   *Signs and*
2. Airway injury   *Symptoms*
    a. Wheezing, hoarseness, coughing
    b. Burned or singed face, nostril hair, mucous tissue
    c. Respiratory distress
    d. Limited chest movement
    e. Smoky breath, sooty saliva
    f. Patient removed from or exits heavy smoke area

THERMAL BURNS   *Treatment*
1. Put out fire on patient
2. Secure and maintain airway
3. Administer O_2 (high concentration, nonrebreather)
4. Place cool, moist dressings on burns
    a. *No* ice directly on burn
    b. *No* ointment/medication on burn
    c. Do *not* rupture blisters
    d. Do *not* remove burned skin
5. Elevate burned extremity
    a. Remove rings, jewelry
6. Dress burns with dry sterile dressing
7. Treat for shock as required; keep patient warm
8. Nothing by mouth
9. Treat other injuries

Position of comfort; Fowler's or semi-Fowler's if respiratory   *Transport*
distress; shock position if in shock; rapid as required

Burns of respiratory tract, hands, face, neck, or genital area, or   *Remember*
infants and children are 1st priority.

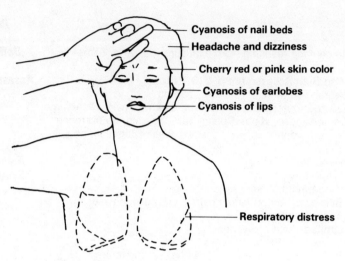

- Cyanosis of nail beds
- Headache and dizziness
- Cherry red or pink skin color
- Cyanosis of earlobes
- Cyanosis of lips
- Respiratory distress

CARBON MONOXIDE POISONING

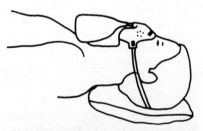

Nonrebreather mask (1-way valve)
Partial rebreather (valve removed)

Carbon Monoxide Poisoning

1   *Priority*

Mild to severe asphyxia caused by breathing carbon monoxide-   *Definition*
laden atmosphere

1. Lightheadedness, vertigo   *Signs and*
2. Headache (mild to severe), chest pain   *Symptoms*
3. Nausea, vomiting
4. Confusion, apathy, lethargy, stupor, yawning
5. Dim, blurry vision; dilated pupils
6. Impaired hearing
7. Respiratory distress
8. Fainting, seizures, coma
9. Cherry red mucous membranes, pink skin, pallor
10. Cyanosis (lips, ear lobes)
11. Bounding pulse
12. Low blood pressure

1. Immediately remove to fresh air (*protect self*)   *Treatment*
2. Secure and maintain airway
3. Administer O_2 (100%, nonrebreather) or assist ventilations
4. Administer CPR if required
5. Loosen restrictive clothing
6. Monitor vital signs
7. Monitor for vomiting; be prepared to suction

Conscious, semi-Fowler's; unconscious, left lateral recumbent   *Transport*

Carbon monoxide (CO) is an odorless, colorless, and tasteless   *Caution*
gas. *Protect yourself* before entering any toxic environment.

Symptoms will vary with time and concentration of exposure.   *Note*

Suspect CO poisoning: unconscious burn victims; several people with same signs and symptoms at same time and place.

Contact authorities (fire, police).

Be alert for suicide attempt. (Follow local protocol.)

Drowning Sequence (*Fresh and Salt Water*)

1. Some water may be swallowed
2. Water in airway produces coughing, laryngospasm
3. Laryngospasm prevents breathing in/out of water
4. Hypoxia and unconsciousness follow
5. Anoxia ends laryngospasm

Mammalian Diving Reflex (*MDR*)

A cold-water (70°F or lower) reflex in young drowning victims that, when stimulated, protects against brain damage and death.
Very long submersions have been resuscitated.
Continue CPR until hope is disproven.

Secondary Drowning

Pulmonary edema may develop following a successful resuscitation.
Observe all victims closely.

Frequent Causes

Limited ability to swim
Hypothermia
Fatigue/overexertion
Injury
    Underwater
    Diving
    Boating
Disorientation
Substance abuse (alcohol, drugs)
Muscle cramps
Strong current or undertow
Loss of life preserver
Entanglement or entrapment
Ear infection
Choking (swallowing water)
Epileptic attack
Fainting
Hit by lightning; motor vehicle accident; fall through ice
Heart attack
Homicide
Stroke (CVA)
Fear, panic
Suicide attempt

Drowning/Near Drowning

1   *Priority*

Drowning: death by asphyxiation from submersion in a liquid   *Definition*

Near drowning: survival from conditions that normally cause drowning

                            Signs and
                            Symptoms

1. Respiratory or cardiac arrest
2. Respiratory distress
   a. Shallow, gasping, coughing
   b. Wheezes, rales, rhonchi
3. Increased muscle tone
4. Tachycardia
5. Cyanosis
6. Rising temperature; low (79°F–95°F) if hypothermia
7. Abdominal distension
8. Chest pain
9. Confused, irritable
10. Restless, lethargic
11. Seizure, coma

                            Treatment

1. Secure and maintain airway
2. Assist ventilations as required
   a. CPR
   b. Administer O_2 (100%, demand valve)
   c. Suction as required
3. Evaluate and treat for cervical spine injury
4. Evaluate and treat traumatic injuries
5. Remove wet clothing; keep warm (blankets, hot packs)

Conscious, semi-Fowler's; unconscious, coma/longboard   *Transport*

Treat *all* drowning victims as cervical spine injuries until proven   *Caution*
otherwise.

Transport *all* drowning victims, including recovered.

Be alert for developing pulmonary edema or aspiration pneumo-   *Remember*
nia in recovering patients.

Be alert for drug or alcohol abuse, attempted suicide, or homicide

Common Causes of and Factors Affecting Heatstroke

High humidity, temperature, wind
High fever
Alcohol consumption
Drugs that increase body heat or decrease sweating
Obesity
Chronic disease
Elderly patient
Strenuous exercise

Heat Cramps

Painful muscular cramps produced by heavy sweating with increased water intake and loss of body salts

Signs and Symptoms
1. Severe leg and abdominal muscle cramps
2. Exhaustion, dizziness, faintness

Treatment
1. Move to cool area
2. Give sips of saltwater (dilute: 1 tsp/gal)
3. Calm and reassure patient; prohibit further exertion
4. Transport if no relief or if condition deteriorates

Heat Exhaustion

Mild shock caused by excess high body temperature from exertion or exposure to hot environment

Signs and Symptoms
1. Weakness, dizziness, unconsciousness
2. Heavy perspiring; cold, clammy skin
3. Rapid, shallow breathing; weak pulse

Treatment
1. Move to cool area; keep at rest
2. Cool without chilling
3. Give sips of saltwater; do *not* if unconscious
4. Treat for shock; avoid overheating
5. Transport if no relief, history suggests, condition deteriorates

Heatstroke (*Sunstroke*)

1; A TRUE EMERGENCY **Priority**

A potentially fatal rise in body temperature due to heat regula- **Definition**
tion failure

1. Headache, muscle cramps (early sign; they disappear **Signs and**
   later) **Symptoms**
2. Weakness; dizziness; sudden collapse
3. Recent heavy exertion (sudden heatstroke)
4. Elderly; chronic disease; skin disorder; obese (gradual
   onset heatstroke)
5. Visual disturbances; constricted then dilated pupils
6. Confusion, delirium, unconsciousness
7. Dry mouth; nausea, vomiting
8. Elevated temperature (105°F, 40.5°C)
9. Hot, red, dry skin turning gray (may be moist if recent
   heavy exertion)
10. Rapid, deep respirations; Cheyne-Stokes later
11. Rapid, full pulse becoming rapid, weak
12. Low blood pressure (may follow initial high BP)
13. Muscular twitching, convulsions
14. Recent exposure to extreme or prolonged heat

1. Remove to cool environment; remove clothing **Treatment**
2. Cool immediately and rapidly
   a. Immerse in ice water if transport delayed
   b. Apply ice packs (neck, armpits, wrists, groin)
   c. Wrap in cold water-soaked sheets
   d. Utilize air conditioning, fans
3. Secure and maintain airway; assist ventilations
4. Administer O$_2$ (nasal cannula, 6 lpm or higher concentration if needed)
5. Control shivering
6. Monitor vital signs
7. Monitor for vomiting; be prepared to suction

Conscious, semi-Fowler's; unconscious, coma (left lateral re- **Transport**
cumbent); *continue cooling* throughout transport

Uncontrolled shivering may lead to seizures. **Caution**

Heatstroke/heat exhaustion signs and symptoms may overlap.
Treat for heatstroke.

Treatment Guidelines

1. To avoid ventricular fibrillation
   a. Do not rub or massage patient
   b. Do not let patient stand or walk around
   c. Avoid abrupt or rough movement
   d. Handle gently
2. Do not administer coffee or alcohol
3. Do not puncture blisters
4. Remove jewelry, rings, watches
5. Do not apply medications or ointments
6. When rewarming extremity, rewarm quickly and elevate
   a. Body heat
   b. Warm (100°F–105°F) water
   c. No dry or radiant heat
7. Do not bandage tightly
8. Do not allow thawed or thawing extremity to refreeze
9. Do not rub snow on affected part
10. Do not let patient smoke
11. Protect affected part/area from injury
12. Do not delay transport to rewarm

Transport   Position of comfort; shock position; coma position

Stages of Hypothermia

1. General shivering
2. Indifferent, sleepy, apathetic; may resemble intoxication
3. Unconscious
4. Extremities freeze
5. Coma (when core temperature reaches 79°F)
6. Death (can occur within 2 hours of appearance of signs and symptoms)

Factors Affecting Hypothermia

Drug use/abuse
Alcohol abuse
Poor physical condition
Disease
Related injuries
Low body fat
Wet body or clothes
Exhaustion
Very young or old

Hypothermia/Frostbite (Cold Exposure)

1 *Priority*

Hypothermia: A dangerously low body temperature (95°F [35°C] or less)
Definition

Frostbite: Tissue damage from freezing cold

Signs and Symptoms

MODERATE HYPOTHERMIA
1. Patient conscious; sleepy, confused, lethargic
2. Skin cool, pale
3. Slow, slurred speech
4. Uncontrolled shivering
5. Stumbles; dizzy
6. Decreased heart, respiration rates
7. Weak, irregular pulse
8. Low blood pressure

SEVERE HYPOTHERMIA
1. Patient stuporous, comatose; looks dead
2. Skin pale, waxy, ice cold
3. Muscles rigid
4. Pupils dilated, nonreactive
5. Heart sounds inaudible
6. Respirations 2–3/min
7. Pulses hard to palpate
8. Blood pressure usually unobtainable

MODERATE FROSTBITE
1. Cold, stiff skin; soft underlying tissues

DEEP FROSTBITE
1. Cold, hard, white, insensitive extremity

Treatment

MODERATE HYPOTHERMIA
1. Remove from cold; replace wet with dry clothes
2. Warm; cover with blankets head to toe
3. Give hot sugared liquids; *no* alcohol, *no* coffee

SEVERE HYPOTHERMIA
1. Do *not* delay transport attempting to rewarm
2. Secure and maintain airway; *no* adjunct airways
3. Administer O$_2$/assist ventilations with caution
4. CPR only if *no* pulse; do *not* discontinue

MODERATE FROSTBITE
1. Rewarm (see opposite page)
2. Dress blisters with dry sterile dressings

DEEP FROSTBITE
1. Leave frozen if within 1 hour of ER
2. Rewarm if thawing

Note

Go to opposite page.

Habitats

Black Widow spider: continental United States (except Alaska)
Brown Recluse spider: south/central United States
Scorpion: southwest United States; lethal, Arizona only

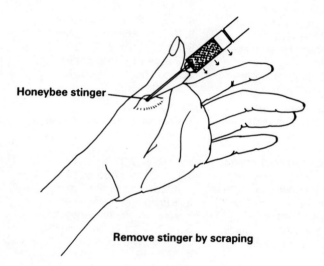

Honeybee stinger

Remove stinger by scraping

Insect Stings

1, 2 (determined by severity)   *Priority*

An insect sting or bite that results in mild to severe local or systemic allergic or toxic reaction   *Definition*

Signs and Symptoms

BLACK WIDOW SPIDER
1. Sharp sting, then dull, local pain
2. Headache
3. Chest tightness, respiratory distress
4. Abdominal cramps
5. Muscle spasms, paralysis
6. Seizures
7. Cardiopulmonary arrest

BROWN RECLUSE SPIDER
1. No/mild pain, increasing with time
2. Weakness
3. Fever
4. Shock
5. Severe local reaction after 2–8 hours

Treatment

1. Secure/maintain airway
2. Monitor vital signs
3. Immobilize extremity
4. Apply ice to bite

1. Monitor and treat for shock
2. Transport

Signs and Symptoms

BEE, WASP, HORNET, ANT
1. Sharp, painful sting
2. Rapid swelling
3. Painful, itching firm white wheal surrounded by redness
4. Anxiety
5. Allergic reactions including anaphylactic shock

SCORPION
Nonlethal
1. Sharp burning pain
2. Local swelling, tenderness, numbness
3. Skin discoloration
4. Swollen glands

Lethal
1. Sharp instant pain
2. No local reaction
3. 1–3 hours later
   a. Itching eyes, mouth, throat
   b. Nausea, vomiting
   c. Drowsy, restless
   d. Convulsions, spasms

Treatment

BEE, WASP, HORNET, ANT
1. Remove honeybee stinger
2. Monitor, treat respiratory distress; administer O_2
3. Apply ice to wheal
4. Monitor vital signs
5. Treat for shock

SCORPION
1. Monitor and treat respiratory distress and shock as required
2. Immobilize extremity; apply constricting bands per local protocol

Position of comfort; also transport insect to identify   *Transport*

| **Specific** | (After ABC's, Poison Control notification) |
| **Procedures** | |

INGESTED POISON
1. Dilute poison per orders
   a. 1–2 glasses water or milk
2. Induce vomiting per orders
   a. Syrup of ipecac: Adult, 2 tbsp. in 2–3 glasses of water; child under 10, 1 tbsp. in 1–2 glasses of water
3. Prepare for vomiting; suction

INHALED POISON
1. Assist breathing; initiate CPR as required
2. Administer O_2 (100%, mask)
3. Keep inactive

ABSORBED (Contact) POISON
1. Remove poison
   a. Dust off excess
   b. Flush affected areas with copious amounts of water
   c. Remove clothing while flushing; continue flushing

INJECTED POISON
1. Remove rings, bracelets from affected extremity
2. Minimize circulating poison
   a. Immobilize patient and extremity
   b. Constricting bands above and below site (per protocol)
   c. Incise/suction injection site (snakebite; per protocol)
   d. Ice pack (*no* direct ice) to site

Cautions
1. Remove patient; protect yourself from exposure
2. Do not induce vomiting if convulsions; acid, lye, petroleum product ingestion
3. Do not give activated charcoal before syrup of ipecac has induced vomiting
4. Do not delay transport to neutralize poison or wait for vomiting

Note   LOCAL POISON CONTROL NUMBER _____

Poisoning

1 — *Priority*

The ingestion, inhalation, absorption, or injection of any toxic substance — *Definition*

When poisoning is suspected — *General Procedures*
1. Determine method, substance, amount
2. Contact control hospital and poison control center
3. Stabilize patient
   a. Terminate exposure
   b. Initiate flushing, airway management, O_2
   c. Do/do not induce vomiting per instructions
4. Treat related life-threatening injuries
5. Transport at once; monitor vital signs, shock

GENERAL — *Signs and Symptoms*
1. Burns, stains, odor, saliva at mouth, hands, clothes
2. Burning, tearing eyes; dilated, constricted pupils
3. Respiratory distress, rales, wheezing, chest pain
4. Abnormal pulse rate/character
5. Nausea, vomiting, diarrhea; abdominal pain, tenderness
6. Excess sweating, salivation
7. Cyanosis, fever
8. Weakness, shock, collapse
9. Headache, dizziness, seizures, hyperactivity, depression, confusion, stupor, unconsciousness, coma
10. Visible stings, bites, punctures
11. Skin pain, burning, itching

See General Procedures, above; Specific Procedures, facing page — *Treatment*

Conscious, position of comfort; unconscious, coma — *Transport*

Monitor vital signs, breathing, level of consciousness. — *Caution*

Be prepared to suction.

Protect yourself from exposure.

Transport poison, container, vomitus to ER. — *Note*

Be alert for attempted suicide or drug abuse/misuse. — *Remember*

Ionizing Radiation Protection

1. Limit exposure to absolute minimum
2. Keep maximum possible distance from source
3. Shield, cover, protect yourself
  a. Wear boots, gloves, gowns, masks, protective gear
4. Avoid contact with contaminated material
  a. Stay upwind
  b. Avoid dust, smoke, particulate matter
  c. Don't smoke, eat, drink in contaminated area or touch items exposed to contamination

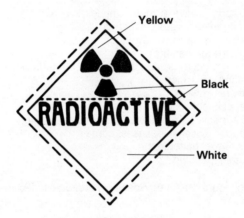

Ionizing Radiation Symbol

Radiation Exposure

Priority

1

Definition

Actual or suspected contamination by recent exposure to a source of ionizing radiation (alpha, beta, gamma, x-ray, or neutron rays).

Signs and Symptoms

None

Procedures

1. Park vehicles upwind and uphill of contaminated area
2. Request expert help immediately including local fire and police departments
   a. If none local, have dispatch call Interagency Radiological Assistance Plan (IRAP) Regional Coordinating Office
3. Protect yourself and others from contamination
   a. Wear protective clothing (cover *completely*)
   b. Use air pack
4. When permitted to enter area, minimize exposure
   a. Work in shifts
   b. Stay upwind; avoid dust and smoke
   c. Remove patient from contaminated area
5. Treat and stabilize patient for related injuries
6. Seal all used treatment items (dressings, needles, BP cuffs, equipment, etc.) in plastic bags; leave at scene with radiation expert or transport to hospital for proper disposal)
7. Transfer patient outside of hospital, under expert supervision
8. Do not leave hospital until
   a. Self, vehicle, equipment decontaminated by experts
   b. Released by radiation safety officer

Caution

Ionizing radiation can't be seen, heard, smelled, felt. It is detectable *only* by instruments.

Do not attempt to decontaminate self, victim, vehicle.

Remember

Radiation hazard labels are yellow, black, and white.

Radiation exposure is forever.

Notify Department of Environmental Protection (DEP)

Low pressure

Prevalent in
• Aviators
• Caisson workers
• Divers

Rapid change
from high- to
low-pressure environment
produces gas emboli
(bubbles) in blood

Rapid ascension or change

High pressure

DECOMPRESSION SICKNESS
(GAS EMBOLISM)

Scuba *(Gas Embolism/Decompression Sickness)*

1   *Priority*

A painful, potentially fatal syndrome caused by gas emboli (nitrogen bubbles) in the blood of divers and others (aviators, caisson workers) who move too rapidly from a high- to a low-pressure environment   *Definition*

Signs and Symptoms

1. Fatigue, weakness
2. Vertigo, nausea, vomiting
3. Joint, muscle pain
4. Paralysis of extremities, face
5. Headache, visual blurring or loss
6. Bloody, frothy sputum
7. Skin rash, mottling, itching
8. Confusion, difficulty speaking
9. Staggering, collapse
10. Respiratory distress, arrest
11. Convulsions, unconsciousness

Treatment

1. Secure and maintain airway
2. Assist respirations; administer O_2 as required
   a. CPR (head and chest lower than feet)
   b. Administer O_2 (90%, nonrebreather mask)
3. Left lateral Trendelenburg's position, elevate feet 20 in
4. Evaluate for pneumothorax (no demand valve O_2 if positive)
5. Assess lung sounds
6. Monitor vital signs continuously
7. Evaluate and treat related injuries

Transport

Left lateral recumbent position with chest lower than feet *unless* head or neck injury, then supine/long board with head and chest lower than feet

Note

Signs and symptoms may occur within 3–5 minutes of surfacing or 1–48 hours later.

Gas embolism can occur in 3–4 feet of water if ascent is made with breath held; also motor vehicle victim breathing trapped air in submerged vehicle.

Remember

Notify ER; patient may require hyperbaric O_2 therapy.

Treatment	*POISONOUS BITES* **1.** Remove rings, bracelets **2.** Rinse bite area with soap and water **3.** Apply constricting bands (follow local protocol) **4.** Monitor breathing and vital signs **5.** Administer O_2 as required **6.** Keep patient calm; treat for shock **7.** Immobilize/splint affected limb; keep it below heart level

NONPOISONOUS BITES
1. Rinse bite area with soap and water
2. Dress and bandage as required

Special *Procedure*	If medical facility is more than a few hours away and local protocol permits, use snakebite kit: **1.** Cut ⅛–¼ in long parallel incisions in direction of fang entry (do not cut X marks). **2.** Suction with suction cup only. **3.** Rinse, clean, and bandage. **4.** Seek medical and poison control advice.
Note	Do not pack bite area with ice.

Factors that Affect Patient's Condition

1. Age, size, health
  a. Very young, very old, small, weak more affected
2. Location, depth, number of bites
  b. More, deeper, nearer heart are worse
3. Duration of bite
  a. Longer is worse
4. Protected or unprotected skin
  a. Bare skin is worse
5. Age, type, size of snake

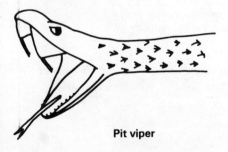

Pit viper

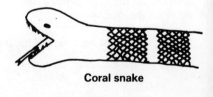

Coral snake

Snakebite

1	*Priority*

A bite by a snake in which poisonous or nonpoisonous venom is deposited in a wound — *Definition*

Signs and Symptoms

POISONOUS BITE
Pit Viper
1. Visible bite (1–2 punctures), discoloration
2. Burning pain, swelling, numbness, bleeding, blisters at site within 30 minutes to a few hours
3. Respiratory distress
4. Faintness, progressive weakness, drowsiness
5. Nausea, vomiting, sweating
6. Tachycardia
7. Dim, blurry vision
8. High blood pressure
9. Convulsions, collapse, unconsciousness, coma

Coral Snake
1. Tiny scratch mark(s) at site
2. Instant burning pain
3. Numbness at site, lips, tongue, minimal swelling
4. Visual, speech difficulty
5. Increased salivation, sweating
6. Nausea, vomiting
7. Respiratory distress
8. Shock
9. Eyelid, respiratory muscle paralysis
10. CNS depression, convulsions, coma

NONPOISONOUS BITE
1. Scratches at site
2. Little or no pain, swelling
3. No systemic symptoms

See facing page. — *Treatment*

Transport all suspected snakebite victims. — *Caution*

Transport snake (preferably dead but intact) if possible for identification. — *Note*

Do not put yourself in danger.

SECTION 7

Pediatric/Obstetric Emergencies

This section reviews pediatric and obstetric emergencies including shock, child abuse, respiratory distress, convulsions, and childbirth.

Guidelines

1. Refer to traumatic or medical emergency sections for conditions not covered in this section.
2. Remember that fear may be a factor in any pediatric emergency; provide abundant tender loving care.
3. Do not let your emotions impede your effectiveness.
4. Whenever possible
   a. Take time to calm the child
   b. Explain what you are doing in simple language
   c. Don't separate the child from parents or caretaker

This section will help you to

1. Identify, assess, and treat the named conditions.
2. Aid in normal and named complicated deliveries of babies.
3. Prepare for transport and transport patients in need.

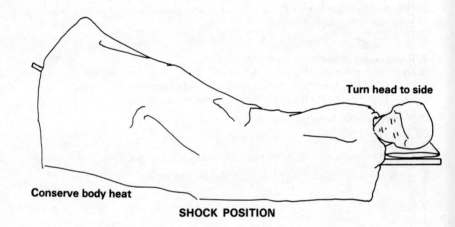

Turn head to side

Conserve body heat

SHOCK POSITION

Shock

1

A syndrome (group of signs and symptoms) signalling the *Definition*
body's reaction to physical or emotional injury, caused by a
decrease in the effective circulating blood volume due to blood
loss or peripheral vascular collapse and the body's attempts to
compensate

1. Listless, apathetic, extremely anxious, restless *Signs and*
2. Impaired or reduced mental function *Symptoms*
3. Cool, sweaty, pale skin
4. Normal blood pressure (early stage)
5. Collapsed neck veins
6. Falling blood pressure (late stage; systolic below 50, age
3–5 years)
7. Rapid, weak pulse
8. Unconscious or coma

1. Secure and maintain airway *Treatment*
2. Control bleeding
3. Administer O$_2$, humidified if possible (follow local protocol)
4. Apply MAST (follow local protocol)
5. Keep warm
6. Place in shock position
7. Treat related injuries
8. Monitor vital signs
9. Control pain and anxiety
10. Reassure patient and decrease fear

Shock position; rapid *Transport*

Low blood pressure will not develop until a child has lost ¼ of *Caution*
total blood volume. Do *not* rely on blood pressure reading only
to determine shock.

Measure and record abdominal girth at umbilicus; repeat later *Note*
and compare. Increase may indicate abdominal bleeding.

Conserve patient's body heat, especially for small children and
infants.

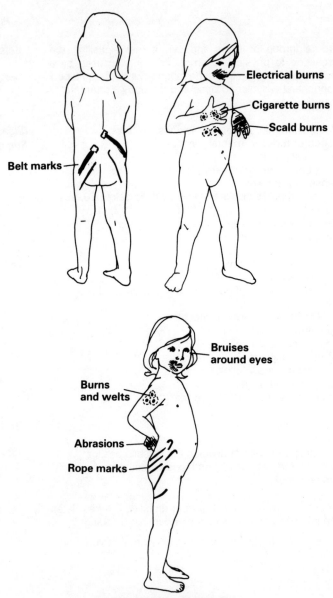

CHILD ABUSE MARKINGS

Child Abuse

1, 2, 3 (determined by severity)	*Priority*

Harmful or potentially harmful physical, emotional, sexual, or neglectful treatment of a minor   ***Definition***

1. Visible old and new injuries   ***Signs and Symptoms***
  a. Fractures
  b. Bruises (new, blue; old, yellow); on ears, back, ribs, abdomen, buttocks
  c. Scars
  d. Bites
  e. Burns (distinct shapes such as iron, cigarette)
  f. Scalds
  g. Strap marks, welts
2. Malnourished
3. Poor health, hygiene, toilet, grooming care
4. Apathetic, fearful, withdrawn
5. Doesn't cry or seek parental comfort
6. History of numerous ambulance calls, hospital visits
7. Parents or guardian vague, evasive, hostile, unconcerned, strange about injury or condition
8. Injury or condition unexplained by history and observations

1. Focus attention and concern on child   ***Treatment***
2. Explain what and why you are treating or doing
3. Treat for injury or condition as required
4. Comfort and reassure child
5. Stay with child
6. Transport *all* suspected cases of abuse

Determined by injury or condition; do *not* let parent or guardian transport; keep child with you.   ***Transport***

Do not accuse anyone; do not question child in front of parent or guardian; do not leave scene without reporting injury or condition to a physician if transport permission is refused.   ***Note***

The abuser is psychologically disturbed.   ***Remember***

Parents or guardian may use various hospitals for treatment for child.

Child abuse has no social or economic boundaries.

Follow local laws and protocol; keep accurate records.

Signs and Symptoms

EPIGLOTTITIS (2–7 years, rare in older children)
May be life-threatening at any moment; a true emergency
1. Typically sick 12–24 hours
2. Sits forward, mouth open, tongue out, jaw forward, refuses to lie down; looks anxious
3. Drooling (a key sign), sore throat, pain on swallowing
4. Sudden high fever
5. Severe respiratory distress, stridor, rhonchi, nasal flaring, rib cage muscle retraction
6. Swollen, cherry red epiglottis; do *not* attempt to look for this!
7. Cyanosis, pallor
8. Fear, anxiety, restless

Treatment

1. Do *not* attempt to look at epiglottis!
2. Do *not* stimulate or place anything in mouth or throat (instant/complete airway obstruction may occur at any time)
   a. No tongue depressor
   b. No suction
   c. No airway
   d. No thermometer
3. Do *not* leave child alone; do *not* separate from parents
4. Keep child as calm as possible
5. Place in sitting position
6. Administer humidified O_2
7. Transport at once; rapid

Signs and Symptoms

PNEUMONIA
1. Acute or slow onset
2. Fever, chills; low or no fever
3. Pain in chest, abdomen
4. Rib cage retraction; nasal flaring
5. Productive cough; grunting; rales
6. Tachycardia
7. Severe or mild symptoms

Treatment

1. Monitor respirations
2. Administer humidified O_2

Transport

ALL above: high/semi-Fowler's; position of comfort

Signs and Symptoms

SUDDEN INFANT DEATH SYNDROME (SIDS)
None; initiate CPR: transport *at once*

Respiratory Distress

Breathing and related difficulties resulting from asthma; bronchiolitis; croup; epiglottitis; pneumonia; sudden infant death syndrome (SIDS)
Definition

ASTHMA (Mild/Moderate/Severe)
Signs and Symptoms
1. Acute or gradual
2. Episodic, spasmodic respiratory distress
3. Rapid breathing, wheezing, coughing
4. Flared nostrils, cyanotic lips
5. Increased thick bronchial membrane mucus
6. Irritable, apprehensive, confused, stuporous
7. Greater problem with expiration

1. Secure and maintain airway; calm, reassure
Treatment
2. Administer humidified O_2; assist respirations
3. Place in high Fowler's position
4. Assist with prescribed medications

BRONCHIOLITIS (2–24 Months; Mild/Moderate/Severe)
Signs and Symptoms
1. Usually follows mild cold
2. Spasmodic, hacking cough
3. Swollen nasal passages, runny nose, nasal flaring
4. Fever, dehydrated
5. Respiratory distress, rales, wheezing
6. Tachypnea (may be above 60)
7. Lethargic, restless, irritable

Same as Asthma, above
Treatment

CROUP (6–36 Months; Acute at Night/Fall/Winter)
Signs and Symptoms
1. Usually follows cold or upper respiratory infection; often ill for several days before stridor and croup
2. Mild attacks may precede severe by a few nights
3. High pitched stridor; barking cough (seal bark); hoarseness
4. Low fever, tachycardia, cyanosis
5. Flaring nostrils; rib cage muscle retraction
6. Restless; tugs at throat; refuses to lie down
7. Greater problem with inspiration

Same as Asthma, above
Treatment

Go to opposite page.
Note

Special Considerations

1. Febrile seizures peak between 9–20 months of age but may be seen in 5–6-year-old children.
2. A stiff neck may indicate meningitis.
3. Multiple seizures suggest more than fever; transport at once, rapidly.
4. Children with prolonged fever accompanied by nausea and vomiting are at risk for dehydration
5. Causes include
   a. Viral or bacterial infections
   b. Hot environment, heatstroke
   c. Previous head trauma
   d. Family history of seizure
   e. Unknown origin

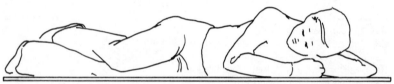

Coma Position

103°F to 105°F

Sudden high fever

Convulsions (*Febrile Seizures*)

1, 2   *Priority*

Sudden, violent involuntary muscular contractions caused by   *Definition*
elevated temperature (fever). They may be partial, focal, or
"staring" only.

1. Elevated temperature; feels warm, hot   *Signs and*
2. Bright, apprehensive eyes   *Symptoms*
3. Crying
4. Skin flushed
5. Sudden involuntary muscle spasms
    a. Whole body involvement (extremities stiffen, back
       arches)
    b. Last 1–2 minutes, rarely over 20
    c. Occur within 24 hours of a fever
    d. Likelihood greater with sudden high fever
6. Unresponsive, unconscious
7. Eyes dilate, roll upward
8. Cyanosis (if prolonged convulsion)
9. Respiratory distress, drooling, frothing
10. Strong family history

1. Maintain airway and protect from injury if convulsing   *Treatment*
    a. Place on low, flat surface
2. Monitor airway, breathing; prepare to suction
3. Assist breathing if required (bag valve mask)
4. Administer O_2 (nasal cannula)
5. Remove clothing; sponge with tepid water if high fever;
   do *not* use ice, icewater, or rubbing alcohol. Place cold
   packs under arms, on groin, on back, or on neck en route
   to hospital.

Coma position; transport *all* first time seizure/status epilepticus   *Transport*
patients

Status epilepticus (multiple seizures without recovery of con-   *Caution*
sciousness between seizures) is A TRUE EMERGENCY.

Age range for convulsions is 6 months to 5 years   *Note*

Special Considerations of Childbirth

1. If baby delivers in amniotic sac
   a. Puncture sac; clear from face; suction
   b. If baby fails to breathe spontaneously
      1. Lay on side, stimulate; if ineffective
         a. Assist ventilations; CPR
2. Keep nose clear with suction
3. Do not let mother go to bathroom
4. Do not forget the mother is also a patient
   a. Monitor status; treat as required
   b. Reassure
5. Do not pull or force baby during birth
6. Handle baby with care; they are slippery
7. If placenta fails to deliver within 20 minutes, transport at once; observe placenta: if excessive bleeding, massage uterus externally; check clamp on umbilical cord on maternal side
8. Transport *all* pregnant patients involved in accidents

High Risk Potential

Mothers over 35
Hypertensive, hypotensive mothers
Diabetic mothers
Mother has infection
Mother has experienced pre-delivery bleeding
Drug-dependent mother
Mother using lithium carbonate, magnesium, reserpine medications

Umbilical Cord Clamping

Follow local protocol
Use two clamps or ties
Place at least 4–8 in from baby, 2 in apart
Cut between clamps or ties

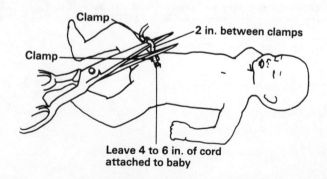

Clamp

2 in. between clamps

Clamp

Leave 4 to 6 in. of cord
attached to baby

Childbirth (*Normal Delivery*)

1, 2, 3 (depending on stage/complications)	**Priority**
Uncomplicated field delivery of a full-term infant	**Definition**

Assessment

1. Patient history
   a. Is this first baby?
      1. Any complications with earlier deliveries?
   b. What are frequency and intensity of contractions?
   c. Has water (amniotic sac) broken?
   d. Is there an urge to move bowels?
2. Examine for crowning (presentation of top of baby's head in birth canal)

Birth Sequence

1. Early crowning
2. Late crowning
3. Head delivers, turns
4. Shoulders deliver
6. Chest delivers
7. Infant delivers
8. Placenta delivers
9. Massage abdomen (uterus) externally

Stages

FIRST STAGE
May last as long as 18 hours
1. Cervix fully dilated
2. Contractions last 30–60 seconds; various intervals (2–10 minutes or more) apart becoming stronger and closer together
3. Slight, blood-stained, watery discharge
4. Bag of waters breaks (heavy discharge)

SECOND STAGE
1. Baby is born (see Birth Sequence, above)

THIRD STAGE
1. Placenta delivers

Delivery Steps

1. Prepare for delivery
   a. OB kit ready; sterile gloves
   b. Drape mother
2. Assist delivery (record time)
   a. Do *not* force or pull
   b. Suction infant's nose and mouth
   c. Assure and maintain breathing
3. Clamp or cut umbilical cord (follow protocol)
4. Assist delivery of placenta

Transport

Position of comfort *with* baby; keep baby warm; transport placenta in plastic bag

PROLAPSED CORD
Cord displaced below and between baby and uterus
1. Indicated by
   a. Mother feels cord slither down after water breaks
   b. Umbilical cord visible/palpable in birth canal
   c. Violent fetal activity
2. Treatment
   a. Place mother in knee–chest position (on knees, abdomen facing down)
   b. Hold baby away from cord with two fingers
   c. Push baby up into birth canal away from pelvic area to prevent cord compression
3. Transport at once; A TRUE EMERGENCY

RUPTURED UTERUS
May occur during labor or late in pregnancy
1. Indicated by
   a. Sharp, tearing pain in lower abdomen, then dissipating pain
   b. Vaginal bleeding (sometimes none)
   c. Strong contractions that stop completely
   d. Prolonged labor
2. Treatment
   a. Treat for shock; administer O_2
   b. Transport at once; A TRUE EMERGENCY

ECTOPIC PREGNANCY
Fetus implants outside uterine wall
1. Indicated by
   a. Acute abdominal pain
   b. Weak, rapid pulse
   c. Scant or no vaginal bleeding
   d. Early signs of pregnancy may or may not be present
2. Treatment
   a. Treat for shock, administer O_2, MAST (follow local protocol)
   b. Transport at once; A TRUE EMERGENCY

MISCARRIAGE
1. Indicated by
   a. Cramps, abdominal pains
   b. Vaginal bleeding, visible particle discharge
2. Treatment
   a. Treat for shock; administer O_2
   b. Place sanitary pads over vagina; do *not* pack
   c. Transport with used pads and expelled tissue
   d. MAST if shock (follow local protocol)

Childbirth (*Complications*)

1 *Priority*

A life-threatening emergency of pregnancy or birth *Definition*

PREMATURE BIRTH
Baby weighs less than 5.8 lb/less than 7-month pregnancy
1. Deliver as normal birth
2. Keep baby warm (cover with blanket or sheet and wrap in aluminum foil)
3. Keep airway clear with gentle suction
4. Prevent umbilical cord bleeding (clamp or tie)
5. Administer O_2 (diffuse flow into tent over head)
6. Prevent contamination by self and others

MULTIPLE BIRTHS
1. Suspect if abdomen remains large; strong contractions reappear 10 minutes after first delivery
2. Proceed with normal delivery
3. Clamp or cut cord after first baby

INCOMPLETE DELIVERY
1. Head delivers, shoulders wedge
   a. Do *not* pull forcefully, but may pull gently; assistant to apply external suprapubic pressure
   b. Suction; secure, maintain airway
   c. Monitor vital signs, mother and baby
   d. Transport at once
2. Limb presents/delivery ceases
   a. Do *not* pull or force
   b. Transport at once

UMBILICAL CORD AROUND NECK
1. Slip cord over head/shoulder to free it
   a. If unable, apply clamps 2 in apart and cut between them; unwrap cord

BREECH DELIVERY
Buttocks present first
1. Transport at once if possible; if not
   a. Let buttocks/trunk deliver; support with hand
   b. If head doesn't deliver in 3 minutes
      1. Form airway to baby's nose in vagina with middle and index fingers, place finger in baby's mouth to allow breathing until delivered or transported to ER

Contact ER for advice. *Note*

Go to facing page.

Treatment	**1.** Treat life-threatening conditions **2.** Administer O_2 if respiratory distress **3.** Monitor vital signs; take temperature **4.** Reassure patient; explain what you are doing
Transport	Position of comfort; gentle handling

Special Attention	*TO CONTROL CONTAMINATION/SPREAD OF DISEASE*
	1. Use appropriate measures to protect yourself
	   a. Surgical gloves
	   b. Surgical mask
	   c. Wash, disinfect hands after exposure
	2. Use appropriate measures to protect others
	   a. Limit or restrict exposure to essential persons
	   b. Provide gloves and masks
	3. Use disposable equipment; dispose properly
	4. Isolate or dispose linens after use
	5. Disinfect nondisposable equipment and ambulance after exposure
	6. Follow local protocol
	7. Contact ER or medical control if uncertain

Note	Keep your immunizations current.

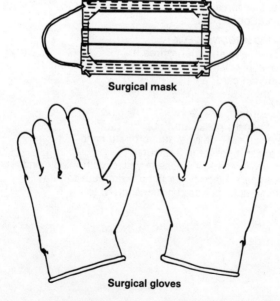

Surgical mask

Surgical gloves

Communicable Diseases

2   *Priority*

Infectious diseases that can be transmitted to others   *Definition*

Direct: Contact with an infected person or with droplets **Transmission**
(sneeze, cough, sputum, blood, body fluids) from an infected   **Modes**
person
Indirect: Contact with material or object containing an infectious agent

1. Determine nature and name of illness   *Assessment*
2. Observe for open or dry sores, rashes, lesions, wounds
3. Obtain detailed signs and symptoms
4. Establish accurate immediate history (especially for child)

CHICKEN POX   *MENINGITIS*   *Signs and*
1. Fever   1. Fever, headache   *Symptoms*
2. Rash   2. Stiff neck
3. Scabs   3. Vomiting
                     4. Coma

MEASLES
1. Fever   *MONONUCLEOSIS*
2. Rash   1. Fever
3. Cough   2. Sore throat
                  3. Swollen glands

MUMPS
1. Fever   *PNEUMONIA*
2. Swollen glands   1. Fever, chills
3. Pain on drinking sour liquids   2. Chest pain
                  3. Cough

HEPATITIS
1. Fever   *SCARLET FEVER*
2. Jaundice   1. Headache, fever
3. Loss of appetite   2. Rash
4. Fatigue   3. Sore throat
5. Dark urine   4. Vomiting

TUBERCULOSIS   *AIDS*
1. Bloody cough   1. Fever
2. Fatigue   2. Fatigue, low resistance
3. Weight loss   3. Sarcomas, tumors
               4. Pneumonia

SECTION 8

This section reviews alcohol and drug abuse, psychological emergencies as a class, and rape and sexual assault.

Guidelines

1. While in your care, your patient's safety and well-being come before your personal opinions or beliefs; don't be judgmental.
2. Remember to survey for other injuries and conditions.
3. Protect yourself and your patient from harm.
4. Avoid making a situation worse.
5. Display compassionate authority.
6. Request appropriate assistance.

This section will help you to

1. Identify and care for the named conditions or situations.
2. Prepare for transport and transport those in need.

Crisis Intervention

To facilitate care and avoid complications
1. Establish rapport, trust, confidence
2. Provide a sense of reality, the here and now
3. Be physically and verbally supportive
4. Encourage communication

Delirium Tremens (d.t.'s)

A medical emergency usually following prolonged heavy alcohol consumption with poor nutrition; may be precipitated by head injury, infection, withdrawal from alcohol

Signs and Symptoms
1. Insomnia, restlessness
2. Agitation, disorientation, confusion
3. Acute fear, anxiety
4. Vivid, terrifying hallucinations
5. Coarse hand, feet, leg, tongue tremors
6. Fever, tachycardia, extreme perspiring
7. Gastrointestinal distress; pain over heart region

Treatment
1. Avoid personal injury if violent; observe for behavioral changes
2. Treat life-threatening conditions
3. Protect patient from injury
4. Monitor vital signs and changes in level of consciousness
5. Treat for related injuries and conditions
6. Transport with assistance or restraints as required

Conditions That May Mimic Alcohol Abuse

Brain tumor
Diabetic crisis
Infection
Head injury

Frequently Related Conditions

Head injury	Pneumonia, hypothermia
Gastrointestinal bleeding	Burns
Hypoglycemia	Seizures

Alcohol Abuse

1 or 2	*Priority*

Health, injury, and behavioral problems related to excessive alcohol intake or use — *Definition*

Signs and Symptoms

1. Alcohol odor on breath
   2. Unsteady motor coordination, impaired reflexes
   a. Swaying gait
   b. Unsynchronized eye–hand movements
   c. Tremors
3. Slurred, loud, inappropriate speech
4. Erratic behavior; impaired judgment; confusion; memory loss; hallucinations (d.t.'s) (danger sign)
5. Displays of anger, compassion, self-pity
6. Nausea, vomiting, coughs blood, abdominal distension
7. Flushed face
8. Low blood pressure (danger sign)
9. Excessive, slow, absent breathing (danger sign)
10. Dehydration, anorexia (danger sign)
11. Grand mal seizures (danger sign)
12. New or old cuts, bruises, unexplained injuries
13. CNS depression, drowsy, unconscious, coma (danger sign)

Treatment

1. Secure and maintain airway
2. Assist breathing; administer O_2 (nasal cannula)
3. Treat life-threatening injuries
4. Protect patient from injury
5. Monitor vital signs and level of consciousness
6. Be prepared to suction

Conscious, position of comfort; unconscious, coma position — *Transport*

Look for signs of drug use or abuse in addition to alcohol. — *Caution*

Alcohol or drug abuse may mask other injuries or medical conditions.

Intoxicated behavior mimics insulin shock and hypothermia; if in doubt, administer sugar. — *Note*

Alcohol abuse has no socioeconomic boundaries.

Transport *all* severely intoxicated patients.

Protect yourself; request police assistance if necessary.

General Principles

EVALUATION
1. Patient history (from patient, others)
    a. What substances were taken?
    b. When were they taken?
    c. How were they taken (oral, inhaled, injected)?
    d. How much was taken?
    e. Has any treatment been started?

EXAMINATION
1. ABC
2. Level of consciousness
3. Vital signs
4. Related injuries and conditions

MANAGEMENT
1. Secure and maintain airway
2. Treat life-threatening conditions
3. Notify police, poison control per protocol
4. Induce vomiting per protocol or orders
5. Reassure if anxious; keep conscious
6. Treat for shock; administer O_2 by nasal cannula
7. Treat related injuries and conditions
8. Monitor vital signs
9. Watch for vomiting; prepare to suction

Caution

Protect yourself and your patient from injury; request appropriate assistance.

Do *not* leave patient alone.

Avoid use of restraints; minimize stimulation.

Be alert for changes in behavior, physical condition, level of consciousness.

Remember

Instill confidence; provide emotional support. Don't be judgmental.

Transport

Position of comfort determined by condition; avoid use of sirens.

Drug Abuse

1, 2

Physical, medical, or emotional trauma resulting from sub- **Definition**
stance abuse requiring emergency care

STIMULANTS (Uppers) **Signs and**
1. Hyperactivity; rapid speech; euphoria; irritability **Symptoms**
2. Increased breathing and pulse rates
3. Dilated pupils
4. Sweating; dry mouth
5. Sleeplessness; depression
6. Seizures, hallucinations

DEPRESSANTS (Downers)
1. Sluggish, drowsy, nauseous
2. Poor body and speech coordination; slurred speech; confusion
3. Slowed breathing and pulse rates (DANGER)
4. Irritability; memory and judgment impairment

HALLUCINOGENS
1. Hallucinations; nonsense speech; unpredictable behavior
2. Poor sense of real time, environment
3. Tachypnea, nausea
4. Dilated pupils; face flushed; rising BP and pulse

NARCOTICS
1. Relaxed, drowsy, coma (DANGER), impaired coordination
2. Profuse sweating
3. Reduced breathing, pulse, skin temperature
4. Constricted pupils
5. Shock, respiratory arrest, convulsions, coma

VOLATILE CHEMICALS (Aerosols, Glue)
1. Dazed; loss of reality contact; coma (DANGER)
2. Swollen mucous membranes (mouth, nose)
3. Numbness, tingling in head
4. Anxiety, tremors, confusion, irritability
5. Increased pulse and breathing rates
6. Nausea, sweating

1. Secure and maintain airway **Treatment**
2. Notify poison control (follow local protocol)
3. Reassure if anxious; keep conscious
4. Monitor vital signs; watch for vomiting
5. Induce vomiting per instructions; prepare to suction

Signs and Symptoms	*ELDERLY PATIENTS (Senile Dementia)* **1.** Memory loss **2.** Impaired judgment, reasoning **3.** Confusion; confabulation (substitution of fiction for reality) **4.** Irritable, unpleasant (hostile, antisocial)
Treatment	**1.** Calm, compassionate comfort and reassurance
Signs and Symptoms	*DEPRESSION/SUICIDAL* **1.** Withdrawn, uncommunicative, despondent **2.** Sleep, eating, concentration disorders **3.** Overwhelming fatigue; crying spells **4.** Loss of interest in activities, life **5.** Recent major loss (loved one, financial, health) **6.** Dominated by sense of guilt **7.** Feelings of inadequacy, low self-esteem, hopelessness **8.** Talk, thoughts, attempts of death or suicide
Treatment	**1.** Protect patient from harm **2.** Do *not* leave alone **3.** Refer/report per local protocol
Signs and Symptoms	*ANXIETY/PHOBIA (Irrational Fear)* **1.** Fearful, tense, restless, pacing, hand-wringing **2.** Tremors, tachypnea, dyspnea, hyperventilation, sweating, diarrhea, pale cool skin, dry mouth, nausea **3.** Poor concentration; feels overwhelmed **4.** Unexplainable or irrational cause (patient report) **5.** Acute attack: panic/terror of loosing mind or control
Treatment	**1.** Gently remove from immediate stimulus **2.** Be firm, supportive, confident **3.** Do *not* leave alone

Precautions for Violent Patient

1. Avoid direct confrontation; request assistance
2. Avoid threatening or aggressive behavior
3. Watch attitude, behavior, speech for signs and symptoms of change
4. Maintain calm, reassuring attitude
5. Leave at once if threatened; protect yourself

Remember   Psychological problems have no socioeconomic barriers.

Psychological Emergencies

2, 3   *Priority*

Irrational or inappropriate behavior that poses a threat to the   *Definition*
patient or others

1. Identify yourself   *General*
2. Remain objective and nonjudgmental   *Principles*
3. Show compassion and understanding
4. Avoid verbal or physical threats and false promises
5. Remain alert for *any* change
6. Request appropriate assistance

BEHAVIORAL   *PHYSICAL*   *Signs and*
1. Fear, anxiety, anger, con-   1. Tremors, motor deficits   *Symptoms*
   fusion, hysteria   2. Tachycardia
2. Mania, depression, with-   3. Dyspnea, hyperventilation
   drawal, catatonia   4. Sweating
3. Irrational, loss of contact 5. Diarrhea
   with reality, hallucinations,6. Self-inflicted injuries
   paranoia   7. Signs and symptoms of
4. Sudden shifts of behavior,   substance abuse
   mood   8. Physical appearance
5. Violent threats or behavior   a. Face, eyes: haunted,
   toward self or others   fearful, vague
                                   b. Clothes, grooming;
                                      appropriate care
                                   c. Poor hygiene

1. Prevent injury to self and patient   *Treatment*
2. Treat related injuries and conditions
3. Transport as required

Position of comfort determined by condition; restrain per local   *Transport*
protocol

Safety (yours, others, patient's) comes *first.*   *Caution*

Police assistance may be required.

A psychological emergency can deteriorate without warning. Its   *Remember*
cause may be medical. Death by accident is possible.

Be alert for drug abuse, poisoning, or head injury as explanation
for behavior; look for evidence and witnesses at scene

Until turned over to appropriate medical or legal authority, you
are the patient's link to reality.

See opposite page for Special Situations.   *Note*

Special Points to Remember

1. Accept all victim's behavior as a normal response to an intense psychological and physical trauma.
2. Avoid asking questions that may challenge victim's judgment.
3. Provide victim privacy from others, and respect that privacy yourself.
4. Use "sexual assault" in all verbal and written communications; "rape" is a legal term.
5. Offer choices for decision making in order to return control to victim.
6. Anyone of any age, any sex, and any relationship to attacker can be a victim of sexual assault.

Rape Trauma Syndrome

Acute Phase
1. Anger, guilt, embarrassment, humiliation
2. Fear of physical violence, death
3. Desire for revenge
4. Physical complaints (gastrointestinal distress, genitourinary discomfort, tension, disturbed sleep)

Long-Term Phase
1. Changes in life patterns
2. Nightmares, phobias
3. Need for support from family and friends
4. Psychological distress, recurring symptoms

Note   RAPE CRISIS HOTLINE

Save, package, and transport victim's removed clothing

Rape/Sexual Assault

1, 2	*Priority*

Physical or psychological trauma caused by forcible, unconsented sexual intercourse or violent sexual advance — *Definition*

Signs and Symptoms

1. Visible physical injuries, bleeding, pain
2. Evident psychological distress
3. Paralysis
4. Hysteria, dazed
5. Hyperventilation
6. Fainting, seizure, unconsciousness
7. Choking, gagging, nausea, vomiting
8. Shock
9. Urinary incontinence (during rape)

Treatment

1. Monitor, assist breathing; administer O_2
2. Control bleeding; treat injuries
3. Treat for shock
4. Monitor vital signs, level of consciousness, emotional state

Special Considerations

1. Be supportive, empathetic, reassuring; speak softly
2. Do *not* be judgmental
3. Obtain a complete history
4. Inform patient what should be done
    a. Report assault (contact police)
    b. Do not bathe, douche, urinate, defecate until examined by physician
    c. Seek medical care
    d. Seek rape crisis counseling (urge this)
5. Do *not* leave alone; transport with female EMT; if transport refused, contact a friend or relative
6. Do *not* examine genital area unless excessive bleeding or injury
7. Allow patient to vent feelings
8. Save, label, and package clothing separately and transport
9. Be supportive; the psychological trauma of rape and sexual assault is severe and permanent; do *not* add to the damage

Any rape case may go to court; report accurately and objectively, without opinion if rape or not. — *Note*

SECTION 9

Special Concerns

This section reviews legal issues, communications and records, moves, lifts, and carries, special care situations, and extrication, and contains a list of resource agencies and personnel.

Guidelines

This section will help you to

1. Be familiar with legal issues affecting EMTs
2. Communicate and record information clearly.
3. Perform standard moves, lifts, and carries
4. Care for patients who are
   a. Blind
   b. Children
   c. Deaf
   d. Developmentally disabled
   e. Dying
   f. Elderly
   g. Physically handicapped
   h. Have specific named needs (p. 271)
5. Locate resource agencies and personnel
6. Extricate patients requiring care

Principles for Legal Protection

1. Familiarize yourself with state and local laws, protocols, standards including those of your service, association, administering body
2. Perform accordingly: keep certification current, attend in-service training sessions, and maintain skill levels.
3. When responding
   a. Tell your patient(s):
      Who you are by name, service, title
      Why you are there
      What your patient can expect
   b. Obtain consent to provide service
   c. Explain what you are doing and why
   d. Show concern for the patient and family
   e. Follow all required procedures to the best of your ability
   f. Do *not* leave patient without care until
      Patient signs refusal form, or
      Patient is transferred to another medical professional
4. Keep accurate, detailed records

Situations Requiring Reporting to Authorities

(Refer to state and local mandatory reporting laws)
1. Gunshot, knife, weapon wounds
2. Injuries incurred while committing a crime
3. Suicides, homicides, deaths
4. Drug-related injuries
5. Child abuse; SIDS (sudden infant death syndrome)
6. Motor vehicle accidents
7. Rape and assault
8. Communicable diseases
9. Animal bites

Legal Issues

General issues of law regarding the obligations and perfor-
mance of EMTs in active service
Definition

DUTY TO ACT
Obligations
An EMT is required to respond and provide service as stipulated
by state and local laws and ordinances.

STANDARD OF CARE
An EMT is required to provide care equivalent to
1. EMTs of comparable training, experience
2. Standards imposed by state and local law
3. Standards required by professional or institutional guidelines, protocols, rules, orders

An EMT may *not* render care without patient consent. Consent
may be
Consent
1. *Informed Consent:* Required from all conscious, mentally
competent adults
2. *Implied Consent:* Assumed when patient requiring care is
unconscious or unable to give consent
3. *Consent for Minors:* Required for patients under 18 years
of age (most states) from parent, guardian, legally responsible adult; if unavailable, Implied Consent applies
4. *Consent for Mentally Ill/Incompetent:* Same as for minors

Legal negligence requires
Negligence
1. The patient sustained an injury
2. The EMT had a duty to act
3. The EMT did not act as another, prudent EMT with similar
training, under similar circumstances would have
4. The EMT's action or failure to act caused the injury

An EMT may not discontinue caring for a patient once that care ***Abandonment***
has been undertaken until relieved by a qualified and responsible third party.

A conscious, mentally competent adult has the right to refuse
***Right to
Refuse Care***
care for himself/herself and for any legally dependent minor
child or incompetent person.

These are guidelines only; refer to state and local law.
Caution

1 | C-MED NO. | SERVICE NO. | HOSPITAL NO. | UNIT NO. | CITY OR TOWN | DATE | DAY OF WEEK | SHIFT

2 | PATIENT'S LAST NAME | FIRST NAME | M.I. | DATE OF BIRTH | AGE | SEX ☐ M ☐ F

3 | PATIENT'S HOME ADDRESS – NUMBER AND STREET | CITY | STATE | ZIP

4 | INCIDENT LOCATION – STREET ADDRESS OR INTERSECTION | ☐ HOME ☐ WORK | CENSUS TRACT

5 | DISPATCH TIME | RESP. TIME | ARRIVAL TIME | ENROUTE TO HOSP. TIME | ARRIVAL AT HOSP. TIME | AVAIL. TIME

6 | VEHICLE TRAUMA ☐ MVA ☐ MCA | ☐ PED ☐ OTHER | NON-VEHICLE TRAUMA ☐ FALL ☐ FIRE | ☐ ELEC. SHOCK ☐ ATHLETICS | ☐ MACHINERY ☐ GUN | ☐ KNIFE ☐ OTHER | ☐ MEDICAL | EXTRICATION (BY AND TIME)

7 | PATIENT'S COMPLAINT | HISTORY OF PRESENT ILLNESS

8 | ALLERGIES | CURRENT MEDICATION

9 PAST HISTORY

☐ ANGINA	☐ DYSRHYTHMIA	☐ CVA	☐ LIVER DISEASE	☐ URINARY INFECTION
☐ ASHD	☐ PACEMAKER	☐ HYPERTENSION	☐ PANCREAS DISEASE	☐ CARCINOMA
☐ M I	☐ EMPHYSEMA	☐ SEIZURE	☐ RENAL FAILURE	☐ DRUGS
☐ CHF	☐ PNEUMONIA	☐ DIABETIC	☐ GALLBLADDER/DISEASE	☐ ETOH
☐ ASTHMA				☐ OTHER

10 | PAST MEDICAL HISTORY

11

EYE OPENING	VERBAL RESPONSE	MOTOR RESPONSE	R PUPILS L	SKIN	R CHEST/SNDS L	ABDOMEN
☐ SPON.	☐ ORIENTED	☐ FOLL/COMMANDS	☐ NORMAL ☐	☐ NORMAL	☐ CLEAR ☐	☐ NORMAL
☐ VOICE	☐ CONFUSED	☐ PUSH PAIN AWAY	☐ REACTIVE ☐	☐ PALE	☐ RALES ☐	☐ RIGID
☐ PAIN	☐ INAPPROPRIATE WORDS	☐ WITHDRAWS PAIN	☐ NON-REACTIVE ☐	☐ CYANOTIC	☐ WHEEZES ☐	☐ DISTENDED
☐ NONE	☐ INCOMPLETE WORDS	☐ FLEXES INAPPROP	☐ EQUAL ☐	☐ SWEATY	☐ DECREASED ☐	☐ TENDER
CAP./RETURN	☐ NONE	☐ RIGID EXTENSION	☐ DILATED ☐	☐ HOT	☐ ABSENT ☐	A ☐ RUQ B ☐ LUQ
☐ NORMAL		☐ NONE	☐ CONSTRICTED ☐	☐ COOL		C ☐ RLQ C ☐ LLQ
☐ DELAYED						

12 | CLINICAL IMPRESSION

13

☐ CPR TIME	☐ O2 NAS/LPM	☐ ICE PACK	☐ LEG SHORT	☐ SHORT BACK BOARD
☐ MOUTH TO MOUTH	☐ BAG REBREATH	☐ SLING/SWATH	☐ LEG LONG	☐ LONG BACK BOARD
☐ ORAL AIRWAY	☐ DRESSING/BANDAGES	☐ RESTRAINTS	☐ ANKLE	☐ SCOOP
☐ BAG MASK	☐ OCCL. DRESSING	☐ PILLOW SPLINT	☐ ARM SHORT	☐ IRRIGATION
☐ DEMAND VALVE	☐ DIRECT PRESS	☐ TRACTION SPLINT	☐ ARM LONG	☐ OTHER
☐ O2 MASK LPM	☐ TOURNIQUET	☐ REASSURANCE	☐ C-COLLAR	

VITAL SIGNS

B/P	B/P	B/P
PULSE	PULSE	PULSE
RESP	RESP	RESP
DEFIB X	JOULES	TECH
DEFIB X	JOULES	TECH
I.V. FLUID RATE GA L R TECH		
I.V. FLUID RATE GA L R TECH		
☐ ECG MONITORED		RHYTHM
☐ MAST APPLIED	☐ INFLATED	
☐ INTUBATION ☐ EOA ☐ ET		TECH
☐ BLOOD SAMPLE	☐ ROTATING TOURNIQUET	☐ VALSALVA MANEUVER
☐ CAROTID MASSAGE	☐ CARDIOVERSION SYNCHRONIZED	JOULES

PROCEDURES

MEDICATIONS/ROUTE

	DOSE 1	DOSE 2	DOSE 3	DOSE 4	DOSE 5	DOSE 6	DOSE 7
SODIUM BICARB IV							
EPINEPHRINE 1 - 10,000 IV							
CALCIUM CHLORIDE IV							
ATROPINE IV							
LIDOCAINE IV							
LIDOCAINE DRIP							
BRETYLIUM IV							
LASIX IV							
DEXTROSE IV							
NARCAN IV							
EPINEPHRINE 1 - 1000 SQ							
IPECAC ORAL							

14 | PATIENT'S RESPONSE

15

TRANSPORTATION POSITION	☐ SUPINE ☐ OTHER	☐ SHOCK ☐ HEAD UP	☐ SIDE		SERVICE	SUPPORT SERVICE	DESTINATION
NECESSITY FOR SERVICE	☐ PT. NON AMB. ☐ TOT. BED CARE PT.	☐ O2 ADMINISTERED ☐ STRET/MED/NEC.	☐ NEED TO REMAIN IMMOB. ☐ RESTRAIN REQUIRED	☐ EMERGENCY SITUATION	ALS AUTH. BY		☐ STANDING ORDERS
SERVICE PROVIDED	☐ BLS ☐ ALS	☐ TRANSPORT ☐ REFUSED	☐ CANCELLED ☐ STAND BY	☐ RESCUE/EXT. ☐ NO MEDICAL EMG.	PERSONNEL		
TRANSPORTED BY	☐ AMBULANCE	☐ FIRE	☐ POLICE	☐ PRIVATE CAR	SIGNATURE		

Sample Run Form

Communications/Records

Oral or written communications, records, reports, and the forms and procedures they require as determined by state and local laws and by the needs and protocols of individual services and associations **Definition**

Purpose
1. To assure continuity of patient care
2. To provide for the evaluation of patient care
3. To record data about an illness or injury
4. To establish a record for administrative use
5. To provide legal evidence of treatment and care

Basic Data

AMBULANCE RUN FORM
1. Personnel on ambulance
2. Date and time of dispatch and arrival at scene
3. Type of run (emergency, transfer, other)
4. Location of scene
5. Patient history and assessment
6. Care provided
7. Changes in patient's condition
8. Time of departure from scene
9. Destination and arrival time
10. Authority assuming patient responsibility
11. Departure and arrival times of return to base

VERBAL/RADIO REPORT
1. Patient's age and sex
2. Chief complaint, type, mechanism of injury
3. Vital signs, level of consciousness
4. Objective assessment, location of pain, suspected injuries or condition
5. Changes of condition, status
6. Medical history, allergies, medications
7. Treatment administered and service performed
8. Estimate time of arrival at ER

Guidelines
1. Speak and write clearly, legibly, accurately
2. Use appropriate medical terms
3. Identify yourself and service
4. Keep comments objective
5. If uncertain, request clarification
6. Avoid alarming or upsetting patient
7. Keep all information confidential

Medical records are legal documents. **Note**

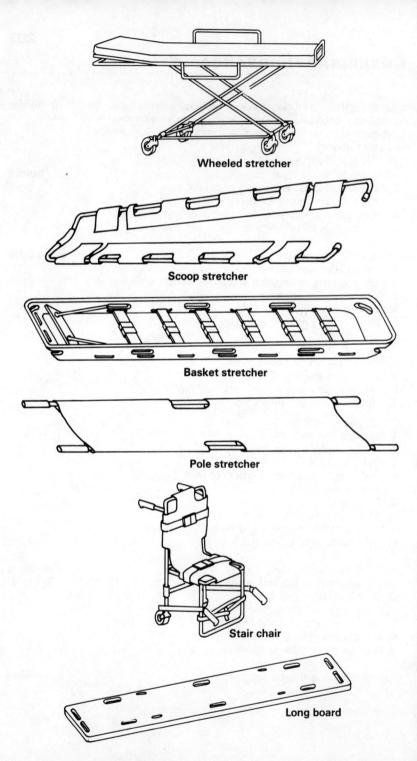

Wheeled stretcher

Scoop stretcher

Basket stretcher

Pole stretcher

Stair chair

Long board

Moves/Lifts/Carries

Techniques, procedures, and equipment for moving, lifting, carrying, or transporting patients *Definition*

1. Protect yourself and your patient from injury
  a. Know your physical limits
  b. Request assistance
  c. Use appropriate technique and equipment
2. Plan the move
  a. Assess patient's condition, needs, danger
  b. Perform required immobilization
  c. Select appropriate technique and equipment
3. Plan the route
  a. Assess safest, most direct route
  b. Clear obstacles before moving

General Principles

Moves

ROLLS
For patient repositioning
1. Three-person log roll   **2.** Four-person log roll

DRAGS
For moving patient from danger
1. Clothes drag   **3.** Blanket drag
2. Shoulder drag   **4.** Fireman's drag

LIFTS/CARRIES
For moving/moving from danger
1. Fireman's carry   **5.** Chair carry
2. One or two person crutch   **6.** Extremity lift
carry   **7.** Three-person lift/carry
3. Piggyback carry
4. 2-person seat carry

Equipment

STRETCHERS/BOARDS
For stabilized moving
1. Wheeled stretcher (uncomplicated transfer)
2. Scoop stretcher (complicated access; spine injuries)
3. Basket stretcher (difficult terrain, heights, water)
4. Canvas/pole stretcher (spare, makeshift, tight spaces)
5. Stair chair (stairways, narrow exit)
6. Long board (immobilization, transfer, spine injuries)

Steps

1. Treat and immobilize patient as required
2. Make certain all equipment is intact and safe; test before using
3. Team leader directs all moves
4. Move/transfer patient
5. Resecure patient at each step in a complex transfer

Device Notes *ARTIFICIAL EYE*
1. Rule out if observations suggest irregularity

CONTACT LENS
1. Have patient remove if removal is required
2. Remove from unconscious patient; store properly; label
3. If chemical burn, flush immediately, remove lens, continue to flush
4. Do *not* use force to remove

COLOSTOMY/CYSTOSTOMY/URINARY CATHETER DRAIN
1. Check bag and catheter for abnormal drainage before transport and secure
2. Transport bag and equipment with patient

DENTURES
1. Remove; have patient remove if airway compromised
2. Place in container and label

DIABETIC (Insulin) PUMP
1. Determine prescribed dosage
2. Make certain delivery needle is inserted; all tubing is connected; pump turned on and working

HEARING AID
1. Inquire; observe if in use
2. Protect from loss

HEMODIALYSIS SHUNT
1. Monitor vital signs and respiration closely
2. Observe shunt for bleeding; use pressure to stop
3. Do *not* take BP on shunt arm
4. Establish shunt security before transporting
5. An open, bleeding shunt may be a suicide attempt

INTRAVENOUS (IV) Catheter
1. Determine if pain, bleeding, swelling, warm at site
2. Check drip chamber to see if line is running
3. Check site and tubing for leakage
4. Establish needle, line, equipment security before transporting

PROSTHETIC LIMBS/DEVICES
1. Assist patient as required
2. Protect from damage or loss
3. Transport with patient

Special Care Situations

Circumstances where specialized attention is required for patients with uncommon needs   ***Definition***

1. Identify yourself; speak in normal tones   ***Blind Patient***
2. Ask if you can help
3. Explain what you are doing
4. Allow as much independence as situation permits
5. Transport with guide dog if possible

1. Identify yourself; speak in simple terms   ***Child Patient***
2. Explain what you are doing; use a doll if helpful
3. Calm fears; reassure security
4. Transport with blanket, toy, doll and parents

1. Determine if patient can hear at all or read lips   ***Deaf Patient***
2. Use interpreter if one is available
3. Communicate with simple, legible, written notes
4. Use simple signing (pointing, gestures)
5. Determine whether communications are understood

1. Establish level of comprehension   ***Developmentally***
2. Communicate at patient's level   ***Disabled***
3. Listen carefully; wait for delayed response   ***Patient***
4. Calm, reassure, avoid frightening, confusing

1. Calm and reassure patient; be there for them   ***Dying Patient***
2. Allow/help patient to express concerns
3. Be honest; do not lie or mislead but avoid volunteering information unless asked; be discreet
4. Continue to care for patient's physical needs
5. Write down any messages you're given
6. Remember that unconscious patients may be able to hear conversations around them

1. Unless indicated, treat as any other patient   ***Elderly***
2. Determine physical, mental, communication limitations   ***Patient***
3. Explain who you are and what you are doing
4. Determine chief complaint, medications
5. Calm and reassure verbally and by touch
6. Transport glasses, dentures, hearing aids, etc. with patient.

1. Unless indicated, treat as any other patient   ***Physically***
2. Allow as much independence as handicap permits   ***Handicapped***

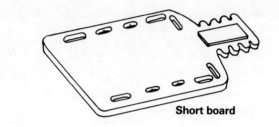

Short board

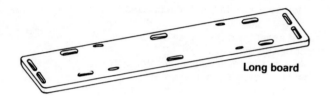

Long board

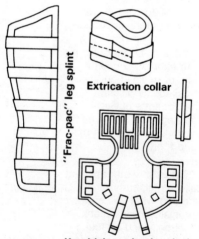

"Frac-pac" leg splint

Extrication collar

Kendrick extrication device

Scene Management/Extrication

EMT responsibilities at the scene of an accident   *Definition*

1. Protect yourself   *Priorities*
    a. Assess scene for hazards to yourself, crew, vehicle, plan
    of action
    b. Take appropriate measures
        1. Request assistance as required
        2. Wear protective clothing/gear
        3. Remove/avoid hazard
        4. Implement an alternate plan
2. Protect your patient
    a. Remove from danger; stabilize site as required
    b. Stabilize patient in place
3. Treat your patient
    a. Treat threats to life (ABCs)
    b. Immobilize suspected spinal injuries
    c. Immobilize fractures
    d. Immobilize; secure for transport
4. Transport

PERSONAL   *Basic*
1. Window punch   *Equipment*
2. All-purpose pocket knife
3. Protective clothing as required
4. Flashlight

AMBULANCE
Access tools
1. Cribbing, jacks, winches, ropes
2. Hammers, screwdrivers, pry bars, fire axe
3. Hacksaws, bolt cutters, snips, knives, chisels
4. Flares, portable lanterns, flashlights
5. Fire extinguishers
Extrication/immobilization devices
1. Short boards, long boards
2. Extrication, cervical collars
3. Kendrick-type extrication device
4. Splinting kits ("Frac-pac")

Local protocol determines scene management chain of com-   *Note*
mand.

Resource Agencies/Personnel

Agency	*Address*	*Telephone*
American Red Cross		
Burn Center		
CB Radio Club		
Civil Defense		
Fire Department		
Hazardous Waste Disposal		
Helicopter Transport		
Highway Department		
Light and Power Co.		
Mountain Rescue		
National Guard		
Poison Control		
Police/Local		
Police/State		
Radiation Control		
Trauma Center		
U.S. Coast Guard		

Index

Bold type denotes primary reference pages.